Health Justice

An Argument from the Capabilities Approach

Sridhar Venkatapuram

polity

The right of Sridhar Venkatapuram to be identified as Author of this Work has been asserted in accordance with the UK Copyright, Designs and Patents Act 1988.

First published in 2011 by Polity Press

Polity Press
65 Bridge Street
Cambridge CB2 1UR, UK

Polity Press
350 Main Street
Malden, MA 02148, USA

ISBN-13: 978-0-7456-5034-0 (hardback)
ISBN-13: 978-0-7456-5035-7 (paperback)

A catalogue record for this book is available from the British Library.

Typeset in 10.5 on 12 pt Times New Roman
by Toppan Best-set Premedia Limited
Printed and bound in Great Britain by MPG Books Group Ltd, Bodmin, Cornwall

The publisher has used its best endeavours to ensure that the URLs for external websites referred to in this book are correct and active at the time of going to press. However, the publisher has no responsibility for the websites and can make no guarantee that a site will remain live or that the content is or will remain appropriate.

Every effort has been made to trace all copyright holders, but if any have been inadvertently overlooked the publisher will be pleased to include any necessary credits in any subsequent reprint or edition.

For further information on Polity, visit our website: www.politybooks.com

Health Justice

For all of my family,
especially mom and dad

Contents

Acknowledgements

I can still remember the awkwardness and sniggering in a Harvard graduate philosophy seminar on social justice when I brought up issues such as HIV/AIDS, the rights and health of poor girls and women, or global inequalities. My curiosity and righteous indignation seemed totally out of place in the context of abstract discussions on equality, rights, well-being and social justice. Until very recently, the most well-known contemporary philosophers and thus most philosophy graduate students did not think the issues I was concerned with were relevant to thinking about social justice. Most of the world's human beings and the concerns of their daily lives were literally relegated to the footnotes in discussions about justice. Justice as an ethical concept simply 'did not apply' to most of the world's humanity and instead, charity was thought to be the relevant concept. Of course, this is a broad generalization and certainly not true of the work of philosophers such as Martha Nussbaum, Onora O'Neill, Thomas Pogge, Henry Shue, Peter Singer, Amartya Sen and others. But then these philosophers have only relatively recently become widely recognized as being leading philosophers rather than as individuals working on 'special topics'. One of the greatest achievements in philosophy in this new millennium, I think, is that these philosophers have brought all human beings within the scope of justice. I know for a fact that I would not be interested in philosophy, or have pursued the argument presented in this book, were it not for these individuals. I am particularly indebted to

Martha Nussbaum, as she was my first philosophy teacher and to Amartya Sen, who captured my attention in the very first semester of college with his talk on famines. I also owe much to Onora O'Neill, as her work on global inequality and public health initially drew me to Cambridge.

Aside from acknowledging my intellectual debts, I must express my deep gratitude for the great material and moral support provided to me by my parents over the years, particularly *after* my graduation from college. What was supposed to be one or two years of public service work has turned into an intellectual journey and career largely made possible by my parents. All my human rights work, graduate education, research fellowships and the writing of this book have been underwritten by my parents, who were expecting and surely deserve a completely different scenario.

I am also grateful to many individuals in Cambridge, especially Melissa Lane, my PhD supervisor and mentor. I owe much thanks to Maria De La Riva, Bill Burgwinkle, Richard Lloyd Morgan and many others at King's College for providing me with a safe, comfortable and supportive home for a number of years. Thanks also to Bryan Turner and Darin Weinberg for bringing me to Cambridge as well as to David Lehman and Larry King for providing opportunities and encouragement to teach.

My heartfelt thanks to Amartya Sen and Tania Burchardt from the LSE for their time and energy in serving as my doctoral dissertation examiners.

In London, at UCL, I am deeply indebted to Sir Michael Marmot for his tutelage and support in many forms. And to Mel Bartely, my thanks for giving me the idea to come to UCL and helping me get there. My thanks to Jo Wolff for providing many opportunities and continued guidance. Many thanks also to the folks at the Centre for Philosophy, Justice and Health, including James Wilson, Shepley Orr and Sarah Edwards for their help in various ways.

I wish to thank a number of institutions for financial and material support starting with the Fellows of King's College, the Cambridge Overseas Trust and the Cambridge University Board of Graduate Studies. The ESRC-DFID Joint Scheme for Research on International Development supported my joint research with Sir Michael for three years, when much of this book was written. And my thanks to the Wellcome Trust for helping me complete the book and supporting the next stage of research. Also, thanks to the Brocher Foundation and the Harvard Program in Ethics and Health for an illuminating week in Geneva. In particular, thanks to Nir Eyal, Samia Hurst, Dan Wikler and Dan Brock. My thanks also to Niels Weidtmann and Bilal Hawa at the Forum Scientiarum, University of Tübingen, for arranging a spectacular week with Martha Nussbaum. My sincere thanks to the attendees of the workshop for a great learning experience. Especially, thanks to Tom Wells, Shaun Oon and Lyn Tjon Soei Len for their time and comments on the book draft. Thanks also to Kaveri Gill, Hans-Joerg Ehni and Lennart Nordenfelt for their time reading and commenting on earlier drafts.

The argument in this book has taken shape over fifteen years. During those years I have been very lucky to have been supported by a number of friends, teachers and colleagues in moving this argument from idea to academic research to book. I must thank Makau Mutua, Robert Kushen, Anjali Nayyar, Sagri Singh, Sarah Zaidi, Tarani Chandola, Sumant Jayakrishnan, Kaveri Gill, Zeynep Gurtin, Alex Broadbent, Dennis Novy, David Kalal, Eleana Kim, Suchi Reddy, Heidie Joo, Anjali Singh and Robert Glick. David Rohlfing, Jeff Perkins, Jeffrey Trask, John Bjornen, Charles O'Byrne, Mark DeMuro and Sean Cross also provided a helping hand in getting this argument out into the world.

Finally, my thanks to all the individuals involved at Polity Press. This book would not be in its current form were it not for Emma Hutchinson, the ablest of editors, and David Winters, Neil de Cort, Susan Beer and many others at Polity. I take sole responsibility for any errors. All corrections and constructive criticism will be gratefully received. They can be sent to healthjustice.sv@gmail.com.

Foreword

Some time, last millennium, I attended a seminar of philosophers, economists and health people to discuss approaches to health equity. The philosophers took no prisoners. The fact that there may be people in the room who thought that rawls were to do with building sites and had not knowingly come across consequentialist reasoning, nor yet be unclear why it was beyond the pale, appeared to be of little moment to these distinguished thinkers. They were too busy supposing what justice would mean if one were transposed to an island ... Finally, in an effort to understand the conversation and bring it to bear on some real-life concerns, I said I was interested in outcomes. For example, the fact that children from different socio-economic groups went through an educational system that appeared to be fair in so far as there were equal inputs, but came out with most unequal outcomes, in terms of educational knowledge, meant that we had not solved the problem of equity. Outcomes matter. A philosopher looked at me, witheringly, as if I'd wandered into the National Gallery and said: 'I don't know much about art, but I know what I like' and dismissed me with a vague mumble about the educational differences probably being genetic and went back to the real business of talking to people worth talking to – i.e. other philosophers.

I was more mystified than annoyed. First, why did this philosopher feel no need to engage with a non-philosopher? Why come to an inter-disciplinary meeting if the perspectives of other disciplines were too ill-informed, too worthy of contempt, to be of interest? Second, why did he not think that a real-life problem was of interest – he seemed to be engaged in highly theoretical discussion that engaged not at all with the real world? Third, how could he be so ignorant of the evidence on education? Simply to dismiss educational differences between socio-economic groups as 'probably genetic' was worse than ignorant. What if they weren't? If knowledge of how the real world worked was irrelevant to his philosophy, might the converse be true: that his philosophy was irrelevant to the real world? This is not to say my view was correct – I didn't really have a worked-out view – but that I wanted a philosopher to engage with real-life concern.

I came back from this meeting and said to a philosopher friend – one who did engage with the real world – I think I'm a consequentialist.

'I don't think you are', said my friend.

But I'm a doctor and the evidence shows that health is the consequence of the conditions in which people live. I am, therefore, interested in outcomes, in consequences.

'Of course you are', said my friend, 'that's just common sense.'

That's not a bad starting point: a philosophy that engages with the real world and makes sense. As a non-philosopher, I'm bound to add – and makes sense to non-philosophers.

Central to Sridhar Venkatapuram's philosophy is how the real world works. His starting point is that Rawls doesn't engage with health. Parenthetically, I do now know the difference between 'rawls' and Rawls – and Rawls does 'make sense' to a non-philosopher. But, as Venkatapuram points out: *Rawls believed that human health is a 'natural good' and subject to random luck over the life course; he sees health as something that is not significantly or directly socially produced so it does not even come within the scope of social justice, let alone that it is central to it.*

The Commission on Social Determinants of Health (CSDH) argued that health and the social distribution of health, function as a kind of social accountant. So intimate is the connection between our set of social arrangements and health that we can use the degree of health inequalities to tell us about social progress in meeting basic human needs. The CSDH argued that action on the social determinants of health, to promote health equity, was dictated by a concern with social justice. The passion of the CSDH about social justice was perhaps not matched by the depths of our analysis of what we meant by it. We were influenced by Amartya Sen's ideas on capabilities and human flourishing. But, as chair of the CSDH, I felt the need for a better articulation of the philosophical underpinnings: why are avoidable inequalities in health unjust?

Venkatapuram provides such an analysis. He roots his philosophical approach in the empirical evidence that health is indeed influenced (determined in the language of the CSDH) by the conditions in which people are born, grow, live, work and age. That is the basis for his move into the moral sphere: *So the central aim of this book is to present an argument that every human being has a moral entitlement to a capability to be healthy (CH) and to a level that is commensurate with equal human dignity in the contemporary world. The moral claim is to the capability and not directly to certain 'health outcomes' or particular biological and mental functionings. And, more specifically, the entitlement is to the social bases of the CH.*

In contrast to an economic view that sees health as instrumental to something else such as achieving higher income, the CSDH emphasized the intrinsic value of good health. Venkatapuram sees health as both intrinsically valuable and instrumental: *Being alive and unimpaired directly constitutes a person's well-being and being alive and unimpaired enables individuals to pursue projects.*

For those of us committed to taking action in the service of health equity, what this book represents is a theoretical justification for the emphasis on social justice. It is a theoretical justification but one firmly grounded in the evidence linking social conditions to health. It is a most welcome achievement.

Michael Marmot
Director, International Institute of Society and Health, UCL

Introduction

I am going to skip the usual graphic story describing the wretched life of some poor girl or woman in some poor country. I am also going to skip over the mind-boggling statistics on the millions of avoidable deaths and cases of serious disease and disability occurring every year. Nor will I dwell on their conspicuous social distribution patterns within every country and across countries.[1] I am assuming that anyone interested in reading a book titled 'health justice' has some intuitions or 'pre-theoretical' notions about the important value we human beings give to being healthy and living a long life. I am also assuming that readers have at least some minimal sense of discomfort about either the causes, distribution patterns, or consequences of avoidable illnesses and premature mortality across modern human societies.

So I begin, instead, by making the rather mundane observation that for human beings to be able to live a full lifespan and experience as few avoidable physical and mental impairments as possible they need to be surrounded by a supportive environment. That is to say, for human beings to live a long and healthy life requires not only having access to clinical medical care when they need it, but also having other things ranging from emotional nurturing as well as cognitive and physical stimulation when they are infants to adequate nutrition, shelter, clothing, access to information, protection from physical, psychological and sexual abuse, and so forth throughout their life.

However, even if and when fully supportive physical and social environments are externally present, the health and longevity of a person are profoundly influenced by her internal biological endowments and needs that change over the life cycle as well as her individual behaviours. So, putting it all together, every human being experiences different types and durations of physical and mental impairments, or different periods of health and illness, and lives for varying lengths of time due to the combined interactions of her internal biological endowments and needs, behaviours, external physical environment and social conditions (Lalonde, 1974; Evans and Stoddart, 1990).[2]

While these are the breadth of determinants of human health and longevity, individuals can have influence or control over some factors, and to varying degrees, in each category. Social institutions can influence some of the determinants and to varying degrees. And, importantly, neither individuals nor social institutions can influence some causal factors. So far, so good.

The centrality of human health and longevity to social justice is so patently obvious to some people that they simply take it as a starting point. This is particularly apparent in the remarkable history of physicians becoming social and political reformers, and even armed revolutionaries because of their understanding of manifest injustice in such aspects as the causes, consequences, persistence through generations, or distribution patterns of preventable ill-health and premature mortality in a population. But such an understanding is not limited only to physicians or to those who work in the front lines of healthcare and public health. For example, Amartya Sen, the economist and philosopher, begins a lecture by stating, 'In any discussion of social equity and justice, illness and health must figure as a major concern. I take that as my point of departure.' He then continues, '. . . and begin by noting that health equity cannot but be a central feature of the justice of social arrangements in general' (Sen, 2002c, p. 659).

Sen simply starts from the position that either in the theoretical debates about social justice or in the practical evaluation of justice in a society illness and health as well as 'health equity' have to be central considerations. However, it is unlikely that I would be allowed to proceed very far if I began a discussion about health justice with a similar starting assertion and especially because John Rawls, perhaps the most renowned modern philosopher of social justice, has seemingly put forward the opposite position. Rawls believed that human health is a 'natural good' and subject to random luck over the life course; he sees health as not something significantly or directly socially produced, so it does not even come within the scope of social justice, let alone is central to it (Rawls, 1971, p. 62, 1993, p. 20).[3]

It may not be surprising that I am more inclined towards the views of Sen and those health professionals who see manifest injustice in various aspects of impairments and deaths occurring in our modern societies. I would argue that Rawls and other quite distinguished philosophers are indeed mistaken in how they do or, in fact, do not address health in relation to social justice. Their mishandling of health justice stems from their conceptualizations of human health and the surprising lack of awareness of the profound social bases of physical and mental functioning, impairments and longevity. In any case, rather than simply starting by asserting the centrality of health to the theory and practical evaluation of social justice, this book presents an interdisciplinary argument that establishes the foundation for such an assertion namely, the recognition of every human being's moral entitlement to a capability to be healthy (CH).[4] Or, in shorthand, a human right to be healthy.

Recognizing such a moral entitlement to the CH would mean that when we theorize about basic principles of social justice we must keep at the forefront the CH of individuals just as we are now always cognisant of the inviolability of every human being, their equal moral worth and dignity, their right to life, or their freedom to determine, pursue and revise their life plans. And, when we are assessing the justness of social arrangements in a society we must evaluate the CH of its members. Indeed, how could we possibly think of a society in the modern world as being just or doing well without taking any notice of the health and longevity of its people? It is also becoming implausible for us to consider a society as being just or good without considering how it is affecting the health and longevity of people outside its borders as well as future generations.

Conversely, evaluating the state of people's capabilities to be healthy – their causes, constraints, levels, distribution patterns, differential experiences, possible remedies for constraints, or potential improvements – will tell us a great deal about the justness of social arrangements. This is because people's health or clinical 'health outcomes' and their antecedent capabilities to be healthy are significantly socially produced (i.e. nurtured, protected, restored, neglected or thwarted) by a range of political, economic, legal, cultural and religious institutions and processes operating locally, nationally and globally. Health and longevity are significantly caused by the physical and social environments – as well as the determinants of these environments – where human beings are born, live, work, play and age (Sen, 1993, 1995;

Commission on Social Determinants of Health, 2008; Robert Wood Johnson Foundation Commission to Build a Healthier America, 2009).

And lastly, but certainly not least importantly, evaluating the capability to be healthy of individuals and social groups will also tell us a great deal about the relevance and adequacy of our theories and principles of social justice.[5] Our philosophical theories and principles should serve as goals and guides to our practical and ethical reasoning and actions. If the theories are simply silent about central aspects of the lives of human beings such as the concern for health and longevity, or they fit inadequately with relevant empirical facts and theories, or they are far removed from how we actually evaluate issues such as the multi-dimensional approach we take to concerns related to health and longevity, then the theories and principles probably need revising.[6] So, because the CH is a basic moral entitlement as well as a source of valuable information – a metric – of social justice more broadly, in both theoretical discussions and in the practical evaluation and realization of social justice, the CH of individuals must be a central consideration; it must be a basic criterion of social and indeed global justice. This is the proposition that I am making and defend in this book.

Justice and the social bases of health

I stated earlier that a human being's health and longevity is produced by the combined interaction of her internal biological endowments and needs that change over the life course, individual behaviours and external physical environment and social conditions. This is not meant simply to be a helpful heuristic model. It is an analytical framework and a phenomenological causal model of natural facts grounded in the sciences of biology and epidemiology. Human functioning, its biochemistry, *is* determined by the interaction of biology, behaviour and external physical environment and social conditions. And any constraints in human functioning, including the ultimate constraint of death, are also caused by the interaction of these four factors. But values or morals intersect with this natural model of the determinants of human health most immediately in the following way.

Of the four broad categories of factors that affect, determine, influence, produce, cause, or constrain ('cause') a person's functioning and longevity, there is something especially and uniquely troubling when social arrangements cause human beings to suffer preventable impairments or to die prematurely. In contrast to an individual who suffers a physical or mental impairment resulting from playing a dangerous sport that she freely chose to pursue, or even the case of a person born with an unpreventable nor treatable genetic disease that leads to a shortened life burdened with severe impairment, there is something particularly alarming when the onset and experience of impairments and premature death are linked to social arrangements. Rather than being sad or tragic, the possible role of social arrangements in the production, persistence through generations, levels, distribution patterns or differential experience of impairments and death is a moral worry of a different kind. It is a worry that individuals have been wronged in some way. It is a worry that relates to justice.

Let me give some concrete, real-world examples. My indignation or alarm is aroused at the role of social arrangements in extreme and blatant cases of injustice such as the killing of destitute children living in the streets of Rio, female foeticide in India and China, or the grotesque treatment of orphans in Romania. Alarm regarding the functioning of social institutions also arises in situations such as the continued censorship of accurate HIV prevention information in some Muslim and Catholic countries, the lack of universal access to healthcare in the United States, the syphoning off of medical supplies from free government clinics in India, the impact of economic policies on alcohol-related deaths of males in Russia, and even in the differential impact of workplace environment on heart disease and obesity in British civil servants. Throughout the world, in every country, the influence of social arrangements on the health and longevity of human beings is clearly recognizable. Such influence occurs throughout the life course of individuals, and in the lives of hundreds of millions of human beings, it is unjust.

Much of the injustice lies in millions of individuals dying or becoming impaired who could otherwise have lived longer or been more able – more free – to be and do what they want in their life had the social arrangements been different, had each person's capability to be healthy been recognized as a basic moral entitlement, and the social arrangements been organized in such a way that nurtures, protects, promotes and restores people's capability to be healthy. Instead, the status quo is such that social arrangements within and across countries thwart or neglect the capability to be healthy of hundreds of millions of human beings, and it largely goes unrecognized as being unjust. Instead, the status quo is seen as being sad, tragic, unlucky, natural, or reflecting the personal choices of individuals.

One of the hallmarks of a good and just society is that social institutions, particularly political institutions, show equal concern and respect to every citizen (Sen, 1982b; Rawls, 1993; Dworkin, 2000). Indeed, the basic legitimacy of a government is said to depend on it showing equal concern and respect for every citizen; without that it is undemocratic and tyrannical. Based on this understanding modern political philosophers have been particularly engrossed in making the connection between the showing of equal concern and respect for every citizen and the distribution of income and wealth ('wealth'). Wealth is understood to be so valuable to human beings and their well-being, and the connection between the showing of equal concern and holdings of wealth is seen to be direct and so robust that any significant inequalities in wealth across individuals within a country supposedly renders that nation's equal concern for all its citizens suspect (Dworkin, 2000, p. 1). That is, significant inequalities in wealth directly question equal respect, which in turn questions the legitimacy of the government. Ronald Dworkin's reasoning regarding this point is worth quoting at length:

> For the distribution of wealth is the product of the legal order: a citizen's wealth massively depends on which laws his community has enacted – not only its law governing ownership, theft, contract and tort, but its welfare law, tax law, labor law, civil rights law, environmental regulation law and laws of practically everything else. When government enacts or sustains one set of such laws rather than another, it is not only predictable that some citizens' lives will be worsened by its choice but also, to a considerable degree, which citizens these will be . . .We must be prepared to explain, to those who suffer in that way, why they have nevertheless been treated with equal concern that is their right. (Dworkin, 2000, p. 1)

Dworkin then goes on to reject the notion that equal concern means ensuring equality in wealth holdings and advances an alternative distribution of diverse resources including wealth. What is interesting and more immediately relevant to the present discussion is Dworkin's conflation of the holdings of wealth with quality of life, and that in contrast to such an exercise seeking to widen the scope of reasoning about the justice of wealth creation and distribution in societies, modern philosophers have given surprisingly little thought to the connection between a political community showing equal concern and the creation and distribution of health. Health, including longevity, is something that most human beings value highly and as much if not more than holdings of wealth. Many people would and, in fact, do exchange much of their wealth for better health or for staying alive for longer. Furthermore, the recognition that most everything in a person's life is contingent on health, including the creating and using of wealth, is longstanding and traceable in Western intellectual history to at least ancient Greece (Anand, 2002). Then, there is also the reciprocal relationship between health and wealth.

On one hand, there is little debate that financial impoverishment contributes to ill-health; the lack of resources to satisfy one's biological needs or protect oneself from harmful physical conditions and exposures leads to impairments and death. There is also much recent literature stating that income inequality, as distinct from absolute income poverty, causes poor health in individuals and lowers the overall health of populations (Wilkinson and Pickett, 2006).

On the other hand, poor health leads to financial impoverishment. For example, a major study by the World Bank that surveyed over 60,000 poor individuals throughout the world found that ill-health and its consequences are often the primary reasons for impoverishment (Narayan et al., 2000b, 2000a). But, perhaps the most important comparison to be made is that while wealth is valuable only for being an instrumental means, health is both intrinsically and instrumentally valuable to human beings.

Being alive and unimpaired directly constitutes a person's well-being, a good in itself. Being alive and unimpaired also enables individuals to pursue projects. Given this important dimension of intrinsic value of health and longevity in addition to the reciprocal relationship between health and wealth, the dependence of wealth and its usage on health, and the greater value of health over wealth, a society's equal concern and respect for citizens should be as, if not more, obviously suspect by significant inequalities in health and longevity as by large inequalities in wealth.

This blind spot in modern political philosophy regarding the connection between the duty to show equal respect and concern and the causation and distribution of health is odd. Someone will surely want to respond that health and wealth are not similar things at all. Health is not like a thing that is produced by a machine at the will of societies. It is a feature of persons, a private good and cannot be produced or distributed socially. Or, some might say, health and wealth are both important. And to improve health, societies need to focus on increasing national wealth and increasing individual shares of wealth. Such views lack an understanding of the great extent to which health and longevity of human beings are socially produced and not just by economic or material conditions. Nor is it necessary or sufficient to have high national wealth to achieve high levels of positive health outcomes in populations (Sen, 2009).

A broad range of social arrangements influence the health and longevity of individuals through pathways influencing their biological
endowments and needs, their behaviours and their external physical
and social environments, with social environment including their
access to vital medical care that protects health or mitigates impairments. When individuals are dying prematurely, becoming impaired
or experiencing pain and anguish from avoidable diseases and injuries,
then the equal respect being shown by a society, the legitimacy of the
government, and the justness of social arrangements must be seen to
be suspect. For, *pace* Dworkin, the health and longevity of human
beings are products of the social order: an individual's and a population's health massively depends on social choices – the type and functioning of economic, legal, political, cultural and other social
institutions from the local to the global; that influence starts from the
moment of conception until the person dies; and it is recognizable and
predictable whose health and longevity will be improved or constrained
by maintaining the status quo or by pursuing one set of new policies
versus another.

Moreover, again *pace* Dworkin, for those who are suffering preventable impairments or at risk of premature death we must be pre-
pared to explain to them why they have nevertheless been treated with
equal concern and respect that is their right. If we cannot, then, as this
book argues, we must take steps towards protecting, promoting, sustaining, or restoring their capability to be healthy to a level that is
commensurate with equal human dignity in the modern world. I will
discuss the connection between health and equal human dignity further
below but, more presently, I want to pursue the connection between
equal respect and health.

In a rare discussion on the connection between the health of a
population and the legitimacy of the political community Michael
Walzer discusses a historical example stating: 'The indifference of
Britain's rulers during the Irish potato famine in the 1840s is a sure
sign that Ireland was a colony, a conquered land, no real part of Great
Britain . . . the Irish would have been better served by a government,
virtually any government, of their own' (Walzer, 1983, p. 79). Walzer
is surely right to argue that the decimation of the Irish due to famine
starvation evidenced the illegitimacy of the undemocratic, colonial
regime. Amartya Sen and others also make a similar assertion regarding the millions of Indians who died due to famines under British rule
(Sen, 2009, pp. 338–341).

Yet, even when people have a government 'of their own' it can still
be disrespectful and show indifference to the suffering of people or

implement policies that are unjust in various ways regarding health and longevity. Various modern democracies showed just such disrespect and indifference to those vulnerable to and suffering from HIV/ AIDS during the 1980s and 1990s. For example, Ronald Reagan, as President and leader of the government of the United States, made his first public statement about the AIDS epidemic only in 1987 after twenty to thirty thousand American citizens, mostly homosexual men, had already died from AIDS and hundreds of thousands of others were becoming fatally infected. There can surely be no greater expression of indifference and disrespect to human beings than not acknowledging their suffering or deaths. Some people would argue that modern democracies continue to show such disrespect and indifference to certain individuals and groups even today. For instance, Brian Barry argues that 'wherever we find groups defined by class (however measured), ethnicity, race or any other structural characteristic that experience differences in the quality of their health, the society has a *prima facie* unjust distribution of health' (Barry, 2005, p. 73).

If we follow this line of reasoning, given the current social distribution patterns of health and longevity within most societies, less than a handful, if any, would be able to make the case convincingly that they are showing equal concern and respect to all of their citizens. Across almost all modern societies, whether rich, middle income, or poor, there are too many significant correlations between social groups with various 'structural characteristics' and the prevalence of impairments and premature mortality. In the modern, post-colonial world indecency and injustice lie not in the causal role or indifference of foreign rulers but in the social choices, including inaction with respect to the social arrangements at the local, national and global levels affecting the causes, persistence, levels, distribution patterns and differential experiences of impairments and mortality.

The tragic irony of course is that despite political legitimacy of governments being at stake individuals and social groups which are the most likely to suffer from high and often multiple burdens of preventable illnesses and premature mortality are also the least likely to be able to participate politically. Illness and death are not only caused by unjust social arrangements, they in turn constrain political participation and agitation for social change. Even John Rawls seems to have come close to recognizing this in his later writings. In his initial writings, Rawls cordons off health as being a natural good outside the scope of social justice. Then he came to agree with Norman Daniels that justice produces entitlements to healthcare in order to keep people above a minimum health threshold. However, in *The Law of Peoples*,

his last book, Rawls observes, 'Yet famines are often themselves in
large part caused by political failures and the absence of decent government' (Rawls, 1999, p. 9).

Rawls further argues that the robust causal connection between the
failure of political institutions and famine starvation also produces a
just foreign policy or global justice imperative. He writes, 'A government's allowing people to starve when it is preventable reflects a lack
of concern for human rights and well-ordered regimes as I have
described them will not allow this to happen. Insisting on human rights
will, it is hoped, help to prevent famines from developing and will exert
pressures in the direction of effective governments in a well-ordered
Society of Peoples' (Rawls, 1999, p. 109).

So, famines show the failure and indecency of governments and
'insisting' on human rights across borders will create effective governments that will prevent famines from occurring. But what is unclear
and indeed frustrating is that though Rawls recognizes political failures and indecency in the occurrence of famine starvation in poor
countries, why does he not see it in other situations such as the spread
of HIV/AIDS in the United States, or in the remarkable burden of
avoidable impairments and premature mortality in Black Americans
and especially when compared with that of White Americans? (Krieger
et al., 2008). Would he have seen indecency and failure of political
institutions in the mortality and impairments caused by Hurricane
Katrina in 2005 or, perhaps, in the cholera epidemic in Zimbabwe in
2008–2009? Why did Rawls only see indecency in famine starvation in
poor countries and not in other situations of acute mortality and
impairments happening within his own country and elsewhere?

The empirical analysis of famines which informs Rawls' reasoning
was conducted by Amartya Sen and Jean Drèze (Sen, 1981b; Drèze
and Sen, 1989). Their research showed that famine starvation is not
a natural occurrence but significantly dependent on social conditions,
particularly the functioning of democratic institutions. However,
unlike Rawls, Sen does not cordon off health or disease mortality from
famine mortality in pointing to the political failures and indecency of
governments and social institutions.

In fact, Sen and Drèze's analysis brought together acute famine
starvation as well as low-level endemic malnutrition under a single
explanatory framework. Rawls' attention seems to have been captured
only by acute famine starvation, and he also ignores the important
analysis of the 'asymmetric distribution' of starvation across populations during periods of famine or otherwise. A reasonable extrapola-
tion of Sen and Drèze's analysis would be that all cases of impairments

and mortality and their social distribution whether related to famines, infectious epidemics, chronic diseases, or injuries reflect the capabilities of individuals and the functioning or failures of social institutions (Sen, 1993, 1995, 1999a).

Readers may have noticed that though I initially identified four categories of determining factors of health I seem to be focusing exclusively on the category of social conditions. Indeed, for much of human history, health and longevity were primarily determined by the external physical environment. And for most of the twentieth century, policies to protect and promote health focused on clinical medical care and on personal behaviour, while also divorcing it from its social bases. I will show by drawing on the discipline of social epidemiology and Drèze and Sen's entitlement analysis of famines how the category of social conditions has very far reach. Social conditions can directly influence internal biological pathways affecting health and longevity through psychosocial pathways and they can also act as 'causes of causes'; the cause that sets up the three other categories of determinants of health and longevity (Marmot and Wilkinson, 1999). Social conditions determine who is actually born and their genetic endowments, how they behave, as well as the surrounding physical and social conditions.

Going backward in the temporal chain of causation of ill-health and mortality of each case will invariably lead us to a meaningful point involving social conditions. This does not deny that proximate, individual level factors including biology, behaviours and external exposures cause disease or mortality. Rather, analysis at the supra-individual level, at the level of causes of causes, provides a more comprehensive explanation of the determinants of both health and ill-health in individuals as well as their asymmetric social distribution. The social bases of the causation and distribution of impairments and longevity are significant and pervasive whereby the causal chains 'run back into and from the basic structures of society' (Hofrichter, 2003, pp. xvii–xxi). Recognizing the causal chains is crucial to recognizing the injustice in the current state of health and longevity of human beings in modern societies. And also important for recognizing the moral errors we make by explaining health as largely determined by individual volitional behaviour, access to healthcare or due to the random luck of genetic endowments or accidents.

Based on the understanding of the broad social bases of impairments and mortality, Sen writes, 'Given what can be achieved through intelligent and humane intervention, it is amazing how inactive and smug most societies are about the prevalence of the unshared burden of disability' (Sen, 2009, p. 261). Part of the inactivity and smugness within and across societies regarding disability as well as premature mortality surely has to do with the non-recognition of the social and political determinants of impairments and mortality and their social distribution. It is also due to the incoherent conceptual distinctions between health and other privations such as famine starvation or gun-violence, or between the analyses of health issues in poor countries versus those in rich countries. This book shows how Drèze and Sen's 'entitlement analysis' of acute and endemic malnutrition ('famines') can be related to the science of epidemiology and our understanding of the causation and distribution of all impairments and mortality in human beings. By doing so, those who have come to recognize and accept that famines are caused by 'political failures and the absence of decent government', will hopefully come to see how the causation and distribution of most human impairments and premature mortality, whether during crisis periods of infectious disease epidemics or other-wise, or whether in rich or poor countries, also reveal similar truths. The analysis should take individuals much beyond the point Rawls reached, and towards the recognition that, all things considered, a government which allows its citizens to die prematurely or suffer impairments when they are preventable reflects a lack of concern for basic capabilities or freedoms, and does not show equal concern and respect. A well-ordered society would ensure that all individuals have the capability to be healthy and at a level that is commensurate with equal human dignity in the modern world, which is their right.

Health and theories of justice

Theories of social justice are useful because they serve as goals and guides. They provide a picture of what societies should aim to realize. But, if a theory of social justice that aims to guide the creation and functioning of basic social institutions is not sensitive and attentive to the profound and influential role of social arrangements in the causa-tion, persistence, levels, distribution and differential experience of avoidable impairments and deaths – especially given the central impor-tance that most human beings give to staying alive and avoiding impairments – such a theory should be considered as being seriously deficient.

Consider that various modern theories of justice along with their advocates have been taken to task over the years for not considering the particular situation and interests of women, children, ethnic groups, mentally impaired individuals, foreigners, animals, the environment and so on. Theories of justice have to be relevant and responsive to the issues facing human beings. Were individuals who experience impairments and premature death a distinct social group, then I would argue that this book is about doing this group justice; an argument for how to treat them with equal concern and include their particular interests in our deliberations about the basic principles of social justice. But they are not a distinct social class; impairments as well as mortality affect every human being over the lifespan.

As Susan Sontag so imaginatively described it, everyone is born with dual citizenship in the kingdom of well and in the kingdom of the sick. Though everyone would prefer to use the passport of the former, everyone will have to reveal themselves as a citizen of the latter kingdom at some time (Sontag, 1978). Impairments and mortality are part of the human condition. However, preventable impairments and premature mortality heap on certain kinds of individuals and social groups, within countries and across countries. Preventable impairments and premature mortality also often follow various kinds of deprivations and in turn exacerbate existing deprivations; physical and mental impairments are often part of a 'cluster' of deprivations (Wolff and De-Shalit, 2007).

Furthermore, it is now well established by scientific research that in rich, middle income, and poor countries impairments and premature mortality closely track the entire socio-economic gradient; each socio-economic group is healthier and lives longer than the one below (Marmot and Wilkinson, 1999; Commission on Social Determinants of Health, 2008). Decency and equal respect shown by societies becomes suspect not only because of the clearly visible and higher burden of ill-health of the 'have-nots' at the bottom, but also because of the ill-health and inequalities in health across the entire socio-economic spectrum. Impairments and mortality may be part of the human condition, but there is much about the causation, persistence, levels, distribution, and experience that is determined by social arrangements and choices.

In light of our changing understanding of the sociology of health, illness and impairments as well as the explosion of scientific knowledge regarding the causation and distribution of impairments and mortality within and across countries, most modern theories of social justice look woefully blind or misguided in their approach to health concerns. It is simply inadequate and misdirected to see health as a natural good, affected by random events, something to be addressed largely through healthcare and health insurance, or determined only by domestic factors.

Moreover, because theories of justice serve to act as social goals and guides, and they are often used to shape or justify social policies, the inattentiveness to health concerns or muddled analysis can directly impede the social realization of health justice. One of the reasons for getting theories of justice right, or to overthrow theories that are dominant and yet wrong, is that these theories have the power to exacerbate or alleviate the suffering of human beings. To put it even more bluntly, a 'misconceived theory can kill'. And there are many theories with blood on their hands (Sen, 1999a, p. 209). Showing the weaknesses of a prevailing theory may be as valuable in promoting justice as constructing and defending a novel theory.

There are numerous ways of fending off my assertion that a theory of justice must be particularly and explicitly attentive to the influence of social arrangements on the causes, persistence, constraints, levels and distribution patterns of health and longevity. Some philosophers may respond that the requirement for such sensitivity and the related accusation of deficiency for not paying attention to health concerns 'runs orthogonal' to the deliberations about social justice. That is, they might say that the value we as human beings give to health and longevity is recognized by almost every serious philosopher deliberating about social justice. Various aspects of the theoretical structures and abstractions used in philosophizing about justice express such value. So, for example, disparate theories will often conceive and present the 'moral agents' of social justice as completely healthy adults who live a full lifespan. Or, in an ideal society known harmful social conditions would not exist unless there were some justifiable reason.

By assuming moral agents to be healthy adults health and longevity are said to be given value because the assumption supposedly asserts *implicitly* that individuals have moral claims to the social support needed to at least reach adulthood in full health. Furthermore, the assumption could also be interpreted as implicitly asserting that health, or at least a minimal threshold level of physical and mental functioning of all citizens, is a prerequisite for a theory of justice to take-off or manifest. This structural assumption supposedly provides, again implicitly, individual entitlements to the supportive conditions that will help keep them above the threshold. And the erasures in ideal theory of known harmful social conditions and practices through the use of abstractions are seen to be expressions of prohibition. So, these and other aspects of the methodology of doing political philosophy are seen to express implicitly the value of health and longevity in social justice theorizing. The assumptions embedded in the theoretical structures or the necessary prerequisite 'circumstances for justice' can be recognized as constituting some sort of pre-political entitlements or even basic human rights.[7]

Moreover, someone raising health concerns in the midst of social justice debates may also be dismissed for confusing temporal priority – that human beings need to be alive and healthy prior to justice being done – with logical or moral priority, that health and longevity are needed to explain justice or are themselves more fundamental than justice. As a result, castigating theories of justice as being deficient for not being explicitly attentive to the commanding influence of social conditions on preventable impairments and mortality as well as for not being attentive more broadly to the issues of health and longevity can be seen to be like someone throwing sand into a highly sophisticated machine; it stops the sometimes highly abstract and nuanced analytical philosophical discussions from proceeding in order for the well-intentioned but ignorant 'health activist' to be lectured in some basic concepts such as the methodology and purpose of political philosophy, ideal theory construction and the level of abstraction at which ideas about social justice are discussed.

Sure enough, hypothetical examples related to health are frequently used to illustrate reasoning about ethical values and principles, but examining directly what justice based claims individuals have or can make with respect to their health and longevity, or how individuals should treat each other in regard to health and longevity are topics not seen to be immediately relevant to discussions on the basic principles of social justice. Health issues are seen as being too profane, too bound up in scientific and economic questions, meant to be discussed in the smaller domain of bioethics, and embedded in the peculiar histories, practices and prejudices of societies in the non-ideal world.

Such views and dismissal of health issues in discussions on social justice have begun to change somewhat recently. Over the past decade or so health has been getting more attention from mainstream political philosophers as a result of what is seen as a novel philosophical problem, namely, the possible obligations to foreigners, especially to those people living in under-developed economies. However, the emphasis of the deliberations on 'global justice' is not on what justice demands regarding health but on what justice demands regarding the well-being of foreigners. Within this broader concern for the well-being of foreigners, especially those living in deprived conditions, the foremost issue is often preventable illnesses and mortality.

Following these discussions would lead us to believe that philosophers already know the right and just social response to health concerns domestically, and the philosophical frontier lies in determining what our obligations are regarding the health and longevity of foreigners. Much of the nascent literature seems to present health justice as being about entitlements to healthcare, and in the domain of global justice, we need to identify any duties to provide healthcare, particularly pharmaceuticals for neglected diseases or indeed, money for healthcare and interestingly, contraceptives to those living in poor countries. But health is not determined just by or even largely by healthcare. It is vitally important, just as food is to someone starving, but health justice within and across countries involves many more dimensions than the availability and distribution of healthcare. Despite the admirable and welcome concern for the well-being of individuals living in poor countries, there is a great danger that the muddled thinking about health and justice domestically will simply be exported to the thinking about health and global justice. Nevertheless, this interest in the deprivations of human beings living outside one's national borders has created a valuable space to discuss health within philosophical discussions on social justice.

Theorizing and moral errors

Theorizing about social and global justice can indeed be an illuminating exercise that has a renowned history and social consequence. However, social justice theorizing that relies on particular kinds of theoretical structures, which makes unwarranted assumptions, or makes use of questionable factual premises about health and longevity leads to a series of moral errors. These theoretical structures, abstractions and assumptions make moral errors by camouflaging and misrepresenting many instances of health injustice. It may be necessary to abstract and de-historicize issues in order to give philosophical theories reach beyond the immediate peculiarities, prejudices and contexts. However, unwarranted abstractions and assumptions regarding health and longevity also 'de-contextualize and de-politicize health concerns as well as mask the agency of the victims of health injustice'.[8]

The use of assumptions in ideal theory such as healthy adults, complete life-spans, absence of communicable diseases, health individualism, explanatory individualism, closed societies and so forth obscure much of the injustices in the causation, persistence, levels, distribution and differential experiences of ill-health and mortality. Importantly, they can lead to the misrepresentation of socially determined deprivations as being a result of personal choice, nature, or random events; they not only exclude the suffering of many from the scope of justice, they also allow injustice to go unrecognized by obscuring and precluding ethical analysis of what are socially caused deprivations within and across societies as well as what could be socially amenable situations. As Onora O'Neill writes, 'Idealizations have their place in rigorous inquiries, but their role in normative reasoning is delicate: relying on them may lead to conclusions that are irrelevant to flesh and blood human beings or blind us to the reality of vile or harmful actions, even when the institutions are just' (O'Neill, 2010).

One of the best illustrations of how theoretical structures and abstractions obfuscate injustice is the pervasive notion that the logical and just social response to ill-health is the provision of healthcare. Because in ideal theory all moral agents are assumed to be healthy, the possible scenario of individuals becoming ill or impaired, as they often do in the real world, is dealt with in theory through the social provision of healthcare (Daniels, 1985). Or, in Ronald Dworkin's theory of justice, individuals who are impaired are provided with compensation for an amount determined by a hypothetical market for healthcare insurance (Dworkin, 1993, 2000). The assumption of healthy individuals and the consequent provision of healthcare, even when broadly understood to include public health goods and health research, occludes recognizing injustice in the broader social causes of ill-health and mortality, in the persistence of high levels of preventable illness and mortality in populations through generations, and in the distribution patterns or social inequalities in mortality and ill-health within and across countries.

For example, in all the many seminars discussing whether Tiny Tim should get social compensation for his disability in light of his cheery disposition, a topic which aims to confront the concern for resources against welfare, I have never once heard anyone raise the question of whether he should get compensation for the possible social causation of his disability. The assumptions do not allow it. The assumptions can also add insult to injury in theories where personal responsibility plays a major role; an individual runs the risk of being abandoned in health emergencies, or at least being castigated for being imprudent, despite social arrangements significantly influencing the causes and experience of their impairments. Where there is little recognition of the role of social arrangements in the causation of impairments, any modicum of personal volition in the causal chain becomes magnified as the dominant determinant, and the person is seen as somehow less worthy of receiving healthcare.

This primary focus on healthcare, which directly follows from the theoretical structures, misrepresents the ethics of health justice as being wholly about the distribution of healthcare; it focuses attention on an important, but nevertheless narrow question about how to distribute finite healthcare resources given excess demand. Such a narrow focus becomes very troubling when the supposedly implicit value given to health and longevity, and the implicit pre-political entitlements within the theoretical architecture of theories simply disappear. Take for example the influential World Health Organization's World Health Report of 2000 where the authors write, 'The person who seeks healthcare is of course a consumer – as with all other products and services – and may also be a co-producer of his or her health, in following good habits of diet, hygiene and exercise, and complying with medication or other recommendations of providers . . .' (World Health Organization, 2000, p. 4).

In such a view health is largely a private good affected by individual behaviour and by the consumption of healthcare. Justice, if it applies at all, or perhaps, the principle of 'equity' would focus on regulating personal behaviour and on the distribution of healthcare. If theories of justice made explicit what they supposedly make implicit about the value of health or various pre-political entitlements, then it would be difficult for such views as these to flourish. Especially because the individuals who shape national and global health policies have usually been reared in these theories of justice and theoretical structures. The misrepresentation and obscuring of health injustices in social justice theorizing is not just unhelpful but actually hinders recognizing and addressing health injustice in the real world. The most troubling moral error, of course, is that the obscuring and misrepresenting of injustices in theorizing actually helps propagate injustices in the real world.

Making the concern for health and longevity implicit in the theoretical structures of social justice theorizing, if it in fact was done purposefully, clearly gives them a sort of priority on the one hand by making them a starting requirement. But it takes away priority on the other hand by not examining how they are affected by what is being debated and decided on as basic principles of social organization. The purpose of assumptions is expressly to fix them so attention is directed elsewhere; and that is what has happened for so long with health and longevity.

The lack of explicit consideration of health and longevity has obscured recognizing injustices as well as impedes being open to new knowledge on how social arrangements, whether locally or globally, harm health and longevity as well as the possibilities for social responses. Why would philosophers be looking for information about health when the assumptions focus their attention elsewhere? Making health an implicit concern of theories of justice also does not produce explicit requirements of justice to keep constantly vigilant for new knowledge on the shifting boundaries between nature, society and individuals in the causation, persistence, distributions, levels and differential experience of health and longevity.

The capability to be healthy

In contrast to theorizing which makes health and longevity implicit or does not recognize them as moral concerns at all, a theory or conception of social justice which explicitly recognizes a moral right to the capability to be healthy as a fundamental value unequivocally asserts the central importance of health and longevity to human beings, and requires social action as well as social vigilance against unjust premature mortality and preventable impairments. Indeed, given the deeply troubling aspect of social arrangements causing premature mortality and preventable impairments, such an entitlement could be foremost a 'negative' entitlement that protects people's health and longevity from socially caused harms. But such an entitlement can also be a 'positive' entitlement to certain social arrangements, or social bases, resources, conditions, support, assistance – call it what you wish – that would produce, promote, sustain or restore a capability to be healthy. Furthermore, as Thomas Pogge argues, in between negative and positive claims, individuals also have 'intermediate' claims to remedies for past harms (Pogge, 2005). All of these kinds of claims can follow when what is supposedly a pre-requisite circumstance of justice or what resides implicitly in theories regarding health and longevity is transformed into an explicit moral claim from the start.

So the central aim of this book is to present an argument that every human being has a moral entitlement to a capability to be healthy (CH), and to a level that is commensurate with equal human dignity in the contemporary world. The moral claim is to the *capability* and not directly to certain 'health outcomes' or particular biological and mental functionings. And, more specifically, the entitlement is to the *social bases* of the CH. This means that given the four determining factors of health including biological endowments and needs, individual behaviours, physical environment and social conditions, individuals have a moral claim to the practically possible and permissible social interventions into those four determinants in order to produce a CH that is commensurate with equal human dignity in the modern world. There is also a further claim that when something is not immediately socially feasible whether locally or globally, the CH gives rise to a claim for social policies that take steps towards making the claim feasible. So, like that of Rawls, this argument also limits the scope of social justice to what can be done by or through social actors; the important difference being the understanding that social arrangements have significant influence on health and longevity. And that during most of modern human history, the control social institutions have over environmental conditions, human behaviour and human biology has been constantly increasing.

The argument for an entitlement is ethical but the concepts of a capability to be healthy, the social bases of the capability and threshold levels of capabilities are not completely ethical ideas; they are also empirically grounded in the natural and social sciences such as biology, epidemiology, sociology and economics. The moral argument is aligned with relevant empirical facts and theories, making it coherent across the health sciences, social sciences and philosophy. The core argument is that a person's health is most coherently conceptualized as her abilities to be and do things that make up a minimally good, flourishing and non-humiliating life for a human being in the contemporary world.[9] Such an argument expressly advances a definition of health that is ethical and rejects others which are focused on disease, and aim to be scientific or statistical. Furthermore, because a person's health is an assessment of her abilities to be and do some basic things, a person's capability to be healthy can be understood as being a *meta-capability*; an overarching capability to achieve a cluster of basic capabilities to be and do things that make up a minimally good human life in the contemporary world. This meta-capability is based on the concept of a 'cluster-right' as articulated by Judith Jarvis Thomson; it is a right which includes multiple and diverse entitlements to goods, liberties, powers, privileges and immunities (Thomson, 1990). Just as with rights to life, liberty or property, each of which we currently recognize as a cluster-right with diverse claims and correlative duty-holders, we should similarly treat a right to the capability to be healthy. Furthermore, the concept of a meta-capability also draws on Sen's argument for a 'meta-right' which is a background right to social policies that aim to realize a particular right (Sen, 1984, p. 70).[10]

An individual's moral entitlement to a sufficient and equitable capability to be healthy produces such social obligations as protecting, promoting, sustaining and restoring her CH where possible. If not immediately possible, whether because of the lack of resources or knowledge, then there are obligations to implement social policies taking steps towards meeting those obligations. These obligations map onto a diverse range of social actors depending on how each is situated in relation to the causes, persistence, consequences, distribution patterns and differential experience of impairments and mortality as well as the actor's own abilities or powers. That is to say, different agents have different moral duties that can range from the foremost duty not to constrain the CH ('harm'), and alleviating consequences of past harm, to protecting, sustaining, promoting, or restoring health capability. Moreover, any agent in the world who has the capability or 'power' to improve the constrained health capabilities of individuals and social groups, within and across national borders, can also have some minimal obligations by the simple fact of their possession of 'effective power' (Sen, 1988, p. 273, 2009, pp. 205–207).

Health inequalities

Despite what it may seem from the previous lengthy discussion, it is not just the social bases of preventable illness and premature mortality or the lack of theoretical attentiveness that is morally worrying. We may also worry about the claims of individuals who are ill and impaired primarily because of the intrinsic and instrumental value of health to people. We also may worry that we could act to ameliorate suffering and disability but do not currently do so, possibly because self-interest makes us unwilling or unable to recognize the points of intervention. In fact, we may be concerned by differences or inequalities in health across individuals and social groups, within and across countries, for a whole range of moral worries regarding inequality across human beings (Temkin, 1993; Tilly, 1999).

Inequality in the domain of health can be bad because it puts people in unequal status; because inequality in health leads to socially corrosive effects in other domains; because the determinants of inequalities in health across groups as a distinct phenomenon from the determinants of ill-health in individuals are also independently unjust and so forth. Our moral concern for the health and longevity of individuals is multi-dimensional and evident across the causes, persistence, levels, distribution patterns, differential experience and possibilities of social action. Unfortunately, philosophers who seek to transpose the discussions on equality or priority of goods into the domain of health fail to adequately appreciate the multiple dimensions involved in the moral concern for health. The idea of sufficient *and* equitable capabilities commensurate with equal human dignity in the modern world aims to capture such multi-dimensional concern.

Personal responsibility

Personal responsibility for one's own health and longevity has to have some place in a conception of health justice. The question is not whether it does have a place but how prominent a place should it have? In real-world politics, encouraging personal responsibility in different domains of life as well as holding people accountable for outcomes has come to be seen as a defining difference between liberals and conservatives in Western democracies. It is a clearly recognizable issue in the public debates about healthcare and health inequalities. The rhetoric of personal responsibility for health was brought to prominence within a hundred days of the new Conservative–Liberal Democrat coalition government in the United Kingdom (Campbell, 2010; Field, 2010). And it was also a central issue underlying the Obama healthcare reform debates in the United States. Many Americans just do not want to pay for the healthcare of 'those people' who do not act responsibly regarding their health.

From the capability approach perspective, individuals become morally responsible for their choices in light of their capabilities, not irrespective of their capabilities. What choices one makes depends on what choices one has. And, the connection between personal choices and outcomes could be established only after accounting for the causal role of biological endowments and needs, and external physical and social conditions. Without that, we would be holding people wholly responsible for outcomes which they are only partially, if at all, involved in producing (Cohen, 1989, 1997; Wikler, 2004; Barry, 2005, pp. 85–94; Fleurbaey, 2008). But, if we can establish that individuals do have the capability – the practical possibility of achieving particular health outcomes – then we would be in a good position to talk about that individual's choices and responsibilities. And even then, when it clear that a person has a capability, we would need to pay close attention to process issues. Holding people responsible for outcomes without any evaluation of the process of taking actions would also be unfair.

Pluralism

The argument for the CH does not aspire to simplicity or any kind of monism. In fact, the argument militates against the simplicity of other ethical and technical approaches addressing health concerns, such as using a single index number for health, making use of a standard conception of a human being or their needs, conflating rationality with cost-effective analysis, focusing only on providing healthcare, or being indifferent to distribution and social inequalities in health. Things should be made as simple as possible but not simpler, supposedly said Einstein. And in the domain of human health and longevity making things too simple runs into great danger. That is, abstracting too much away from the reality of the daily lives and concerns of human beings and the global human community to the point of being irrelevant, or erasing too much of the complexity of the causes, constraints, persistence, distribution patterns, consequences and possible remedies of preventable ill-health and mortality runs the risk of obfuscating injustice and thereby, tolerating or exacerbating it.

What I am presenting is a plural account of health justice under the guise of a single moral entitlement to a capability to be healthy.[11] The right to the CH is a right to a cluster of diverse entitlements. This is not the place to explain or defend value pluralism, and it will have to suffice for me to say that value pluralism is an intrinsic part of the capabilities approach (Qizilbash, 1997; Alkire, 2002; Wolff and De-Shalit, 2007). The argument I am making also is not something fundamentally original, too complex and unworkable, or all-encompassing. The argument stands on the shoulders of giants; it unabashedly builds on the work of others. It will become plain that there has been a long-standing international movement to recognize health as an assessment of abilities to function in the world. We also already recognize complex cluster-rights that I present here as a meta-capability. We already recognize that multiple actors can have obligations correlative to a given moral entitlement or legal right; that these obligations can be of different kinds; and that each actor can be obligated at different times with less or more stringency.

What can be seen as original, referring back to the initial proposition about the centrality of health to social justice, is that I ground the entitlement to a health capability in our shared values of human freedom and in showing respect for the equal dignity of every human being; both these values are central components or 'rock bottom' values of liberal social justice. The capability to be healthy is a kind of freedom, which is intrinsically and instrumentally valuable, and which almost every human being and society is likely to value, albeit for a wide variety of reasons. At the same time, showing respect for the equal dignity of human beings means ensuring every individual has the real opportunity to be healthy, to live a life of activity and opportunity worthy of the dignity of a human being.

The CH is a minimal account of well-being that is commensurate with equal human dignity in the modern world. Therefore, by linking a person's CH to her freedom and equal human dignity, health is grounded in both the fundamental values of liberty and equality, and made a central concern of social justice. The importance of an argument about health claims such as this appealing to justice, as opposed to beneficence, economic growth or national interest and security, is to claim priority over all other social values and goals (Nagel, 1997). Health injustice as a particular kind of social injustice is not just a bad, sad or tragic situation; it should not be tolerated and is to be avoided to the greatest extent possible. There is no greater ought for social action. So, indeed, much is at stake in the following argument that brings together human health and longevity, the concept of a capability to be healthy, and an approach to social justice that guarantees the social bases of capabilities.

The capabilities approach

This argument for the moral entitlement to the social bases of a CH extends the capabilities approach (CA) conceived and championed by Amartya Sen, and developed differently by Martha Nussbaum, into the domain of human health. I say the domain of health because it is not just an extension into healthcare policy or health sector policy but into all social deliberations and policies that affect health. Ensuring that individuals have the capability to be healthy requires not only getting healthcare institutions right but also getting right the much broader social arrangements that influence the causation, persistence, distribution, levels and experience of health and longevity. The present argument brings together most immediately concepts and debates in the philosophy of medicine and health, epidemiology, sociology, public health and political philosophy in order to put forward an interdisciplinary argument. This is an exercise in applied and practical philosophy. And it is meant to be an argument that would interest individuals beyond academic philosophers. Like the CA in general, the CH argument is meant to practically guide real-world public policy and social action.

It seems, however, that the CA is many things to many people and is continuing to evolve rapidly. Until about ten years ago, the CA was what Amartya Sen or Martha Nussbaum said it was in their latest publication. Now, there are numerous advocates of the CA around the world, with some developing their own particular variations. There is also no set text for the CA (so far), and unfortunately, some variations and interpretations are erroneous.[12] In order not to further contribute to possible confusion, in this book the CA is recognized as (1) an analytical, evaluative framework for making inter-personal comparisons of well-being or advantage for public policy purposes; (2) a method of measuring and assessing the state of a nation or populations; (3) a critique of the dominant conceptions of social justice in twentieth-century Anglo-American philosophy; and (4) an approach or partial theory of social justice and social development (Sen, 1982a, 1992a; Nussbaum and Sen, 1993; Nussbaum et al., 1995; Sen, 1997; Nussbaum, 1999; Sen, 1999a; Nussbaum, 2000b, 2006; Basu et al., 2009; Sen, 2009).

Given all these different uses of the CA, its diverse application across many disciplines, and for bridging theory and practice or morality and politics, the CA has been understandably described as an 'intellectual movement'. It also serves as a 'counter-theory' to the dominant theories in different fields of enquiry and practice. Nevertheless, whatever their setting or purpose, advocates of the CA champion the central idea that the well-being of individuals is *best* reflected in and promoted through their capabilities to be and doing certain things in pursuing their life plans. This is in contrast to alternative foci such as a person's resources (income and wealth, primary goods) and mental welfare (utility, preferences, happiness), a country's aggregate economic indicators such as Gross Domestic Product (GDP) and Gross National Product (GNP), or even population averages such as GDP or GNP per capita. And, it is worth mentioning because of its particular relevance to the argument of this book, the CA's initial line of reasoning in the domain of health is that we should be evaluating the health capabilities of people and not primarily the size of financial investments or spending in the health sector, total or average household spending on healthcare, average health indicators of the population, or how people feel about their own health. Probably the best evidence of how misdirected it is to evaluate the health of individuals and of a national population by the size of its healthcare spending is to look at the size of healthcare spending in the United States, the health of its population, and then compare with other countries (Farley, 2009; Lobb, 2009). The United States also provides a very good illustration of how national averages of health measures can hide substantial inequalities in health among social groups (Rogot et al., 1992; Sorlie et al., 1992; Murray et al., 1998; Lin et al., 2003; Asada, 2005; Kawachi et al., 2005).

In academic philosophy the CA is viewed as one among a range of ethical schools competing to establish the right understanding of liberal and egalitarian social justice. Different theories aim to socially guarantee or 'distribute' various things such as individual liberties, resources such as income, welfare, opportunities for advantage, capabilities and so forth. And currently, the CA is seen as ascendant against theories which focus on distributing resources or focus on some aspect of mental states such as satisfaction or happiness. Yet, as the saying goes, every new faith soon becomes the old orthodoxy. For now, the CA is the new faith and until recently, it was Rawls' theory of justice as fairness. And the orthodoxy which Rawls wanted to overthrow was utilitarianism. Welfarist theories are various permutations of utilitarianism which focus on such things as utility, preferences or happiness but can also focus on objective measurements such as length of lifespan. The central idea, however, is that the right thing to do will be that which maximizes welfare. Despite its pervasive influence on public policy, particularly through its influence in economics, utilitarianism has long been seen as morally deficient in academic political philosophy.

Part of the significance of Rawls' accomplishment was to offer a plausible alternative. In any case, utilitarianism is very much alive in the real world, and nowhere more kicking than in public health and health policy, particularly in developing countries. It is largely taken for granted that a health policy aims to maximize whether it is the number of vaccinations, sterilizations, disease cases averted, Quality Adjusted Life Years (QALYs), Disability Adjusted Life Years (DALYS), or something else. The extension of the CA into the domain of health in academic philosophical debates may rightly focus on the subtle differences between Rawlsian primary goods versus capabilities, but in the real world, the orthodoxy that requires confronting is that of maximizing health or health improvement.

While it may initially seem like heresy, part of the aim of this book is to show why maximization of health outcomes may not always be what justice requires. Equal concern and respect for individuals requires that we evaluate and respond accordingly to the multiple dimensions of the capability to be healthy – the causes, persistence, social distribution, levels and differential experience of impairments and mortality. Alleviating injustice may require something different than efficiency (i.e. maximizing levels of health outcomes).

Despite the CA's full engagement with its theoretical rivals regarding the right conception of social justice in academic discussions, the CA is also a field of praxis and an agenda for practical social change. There is a focus on capabilities because they are seen to be the correct ethical goods of social justice and because they are the means for social development; human capabilities are both the means and the normative goals. The empirical assertion is that protecting, nurturing and restoring people's capabilities will causally produce more individual and social well-being (Sen, 1999a, ch. 2). Because of its ethical and empirical assertions, over the past thirty years since its initial articulation, the CA has had significant influence in numerous fields including welfare economics, political philosophy and social development planning and policy.

Initially, the CA was influential in international development communities including institutions such the World Bank and United Nations agencies such as the UN Development Programme. Increasingly, the CA's influence is now also becoming visible in the public deliberations and policies of high income countries. For example, in European countries the CA is being applied in a variety of domains including economic policies,[13] social equality policies,[14] health reviews[15] and even political party manifestos.[16]

Health and the capabilities approach

In Sen's discussions on the basic capabilities that he thinks most societies will find valuable or in Nussbaum's ten central human capabilities (CHCs), health capability or capabilities are present and prominent.[17] But they are too under-described by both individuals. Indeed, health capabilities are probably less ambiguous and less neglected in the CA literature than other capabilities that could also be considered basic such as capabilities related to education, or to political participation. The general schematic nature of capabilities in the literature, even Nussbaum's ten CHCs, may be understandable given Sen and Nussbaum are advancing a general approach or theory to social justice rather than one particular capability. At the same time, Nussbaum rightly recognizes that health institutions are equipped with necessary but often abused powers of coercion and paternalism. And, even international human rights law allows states to limit liberty and derogate from human rights law in the name of public health.

For many reasons – the abuse of coercive powers in the name of health policy and public health, the gravity of situations where social arrangements are causing premature mortality and ill-health, the centrality of health to people's everyday living and future plans, and the astounding epidemiological research on the psychosocial determinants of ill-health and the social gradient in health – the CA cannot continue to be schematic regarding health capability; providing only a rough outline of a health capability is unsatisfactory and urgently in need of fleshing out. This becomes even more obvious when we find how health has been given so much more focused attention by the competing approaches to social justice (Broome, 2006; Daniels, 2008; Segall, 2009). Or, is it that the other approaches are able to do so because they have a simpler view of health and health justice? CA advocates may indeed believe that welfare or resource theories have it completely wrong regarding health, but we have yet to provide a clear argument for how the CA addresses health concerns and does it better than the alternatives.

Indeed, there have been some nascent attempts over the years, and recently Jennifer Prah Ruger presented a forceful case for applying a health capability paradigm to health policy. She has put down an important marker in the debates on behalf of the CA. The scope of her argument, however, is confined to healthcare policy and not to the broader social arrangements that affect health or the multi-dimensional aspects of human health and longevity (Ruger, 2010). Health justice requires that we get more than healthcare policy right. We must get the social arrangements, the social policy, for health right. There is still much to do in the CA regarding theorizing health justice.

A 'general theory' of health and social justice needs to describe what health is, how it is created and distributed, and why it is valuable to human beings. It should also be able to identify what claims and obligations individuals have in regard to their health and the implications for the rights and duties of other agents. And, it should hopefully help guide action at the policy level and in the face of difficult circumstances. For the sake of simplicity, the capacity to describe what health is and how it is created and distributed can be thought of as the descriptive capacities of such a theory. Its capacity to guide an ethical social response to ill-health and inequalities in health across individuals and groups can be thought of as its normative capacities. The argument for an entitlement to a CH presented in this book has many of these capacities, and much more. But the argument is not presented as a general theory because it is insufficient to be a theory by itself. And it is unlikely that it could be a full theory even if it relied even more heavily on the CA than it does already. That is, fleshing out a health capability within a general theory of capabilities would be one way to produce a theory of health and social justice. There is quite a respectable tradition of extending or amending theories of justice in response to specific concerns (Beitz, 1975; Daniels, 1985; Pogge, 1989; Daniels, 2008). But such an option is unavailable, at least for now. On the one hand, Sen rejects the need for 'transcendental theories' to do justice, implying that the CA is not intended to be one those comprehensive theories (Sen, 2006; Sen, 2009).

Moreover, Sen is also very clear that capabilities, though a significant part of justice, do not constitute the entirety of justice (Sen, 2010). Capabilities are seen as the basis of a measure of overall individual advantages and for making interpersonal comparisons of overall advantages, not measuring justice (Sen, 2010, p. 243). Sen has also recently identified various open textured principles such as priority of liberty, fairness, process, objectivity and impartiality as being central to realizing justice. He provides no formal, defined theory, and instead advocates a more contextual and 'comparative approach' (Sen, 2009).

On the other hand, Nussbaum asserts that her version of the CA is only a 'partial' or incomplete theory of justice. Her argument for ensuring ten CHCs says nothing about inequalities in these capabilities above certain sufficiency thresholds or about the pursuit of other social goals along side ensuring the ten central human capabilities; it is meant to be a minimally sufficient conception of social justice (Nussbaum, 2006, pp. 70–71). So in either case, extending the CA in its present form to include health concerns will not deliver a full theory of health and social justice. And much work will remain to be done even after what is presented in this book. Therefore, what is presented here can be understood as (i) articulating an argument from the capabilities approach for the capability to be healthy; (ii) a framework and ethical justification for a human entitlement to the capability to be healthy ('the human right to health'); and (iii) an entitlement that stands at the centre of a theory of health justice with a more complete theory in the process of being developed.

I should say at the outset that it would be misguided to interpret the present CH argument as either advocating the forcing of individuals to be healthy, or as making scientifically ill-informed arguments for entitlements to fantastic, impossible or ideal health achievements. The spectre of perfectionism or the infeasibility critique directed against the CA can also be as easily and mistakenly hurled against the argument for the CH. To reiterate, the present argument is for the entitlement to the *social bases* of the CH, what is possible through public policy and social choice. It also reflects a continual awareness of two dimensions.

On the one hand, the argument recognizes the normative importance of individual choice and responsibility in liberal theory. But the respect for individual agency is set against the background of our most current sociological understandings of the links between agency and (global) social structures. It is also informed by the agency-structure debates in specific relation to health issues (Turner, 2004). On the other hand, the argument also reflects an awareness of the most current scientific developments in the health sciences such as epidemiology while taking a critical view of the parameters, methodologies and social practices of scientific research (Weed, 2001; Trostle, 2004; Cribb, 2005; Venkatapuram, 2006; Rothman et al., 2008).

Outline of the argument and book

The book is organized into three parts. Part I advances a conception of health as capability, and presents a theory of causation and distribution of health capabilities. Part II reviews capabilities theory and presents the argument for the CH. Part III reviews five alternative ethical approaches to health claims as well as considers the implications of the CH argument for dealing with groups and global justice. The three parts of the argument are mutually reinforcing, and the entire argument is inter-disciplinary. Applied philosophy necessarily has to be interdisciplinary as it applies philosophical scrutiny to a particular subject that can have its own distinct assumptions, goals and methodology. Such an endeavour is particularly complicated when philosophical scrutiny takes aim at the natural or biological sciences as they are often perceived and presented to be outside the domain of values.

The arguments presented here will hopefully help create some common understanding across the natural and social sciences as well as ethics on some issues including the concept of human health, how it is caused and distributed, and what the ethical social response should be to the causes, persistence, absolute levels, distribution patterns, differential experience and relative differences in health capability across individuals, groups and national populations.

If it is helpful, Part I may be categorized as arguments within the sub-disciplines of philosophy of health, medicine and epidemiology. Parts II and III are arguments in political philosophy that are situated against the background debates on whether the focal point of distributive justice should be on individual welfare, resources or capabilities. The largely descriptive or empirical arguments of Part I are presented in conjunction with the normative argument for a moral entitlement to a CH in Parts II and III because they provide independent support for the CH; they provide external validation of the stability of the argument. Part I establishes independently outside of capabilities theory the coherence of understanding health as a capability and of the science behind the social bases of a health capability. This is important because there is a fundamental issue as to how one proves or justifies that one theory of justice is better than another if the core of each is based on an incommensurable value with another. By providing independent support from philosophy of health and the science of epidemiology, I am showing how the capabilities approach to health, and the argument for the CH more specifically, are plausible and have stability as there is inter-theoretic coherence across relevant disciplines and state-of-the-art knowledge on health and longevity.

Part I

In Chapter 1, I present a theory of human health as a CH, or more specifically, an overarching 'meta-capability'. I advance a conception of health as being an assessment of a person's capability to achieve, exercise or express ('achieve') a cluster of basic and inter-related capabilities and functionings; a meta-capability. I arrive at the notion of health as a capability to achieve a cluster of basic capabilities through first rejecting the incoherent though dominant view of health as the absence of disease or species typical functioning. This classic and purportedly scientific account initially advocated by Christopher Boorse in the 1970s has numerous flaws which are reviewed. Eschewing the 'naturalistic', scientific, or objective path to a definition of human health, I instead put forward a conception of health as the assessment of a cluster of basic capabilities. This conception is indebted to Lennart Nordenfelt's theory of health, which posits health as the ability to achieve a set of 'vital goals'. But because Nordenfelt's theory relies too much on subjective preferences and allows for cultural relativism, I transform Nordenfelt's conception of health into a minimum conception of vital goals that is applicable across the human species. This is done by replacing the empty set of vital goals in Nordenfelt's conception with Nussbaum's account of central human capabilities (CHCs), or activities and opportunities that constitute a life with minimal human dignity.

Nussbaum also offers reasoning to understand these basic capabilities as pre-political moral entitlements; claims to social support for exercising these basic capabilities are a source of basic political principles guiding social organization. So rather than the local culture or social environment defining vital goals, as in Nordenfelt's original theory, the claims to central human capabilities shape the social environment.

In Chapter 2, I review the state of the research in epidemiology on the social causation and distribution of disease, and advance a 'unified' theory of causation and distribution of health capability. The theory I advocate is informed by the 'entitlement theory' of famines. This is the same theory which is referred to by Rawls, that was developed in the field of development economics, and which gave rise to the concept of capabilities. Applying the entitlement theory to epidemiology conceptually integrates the four causal categories of factors, which include individual biology, physical exposures, social conditions and individual agency (skills and choices).

Although in Chapter 1 I advocate a conception of health as capability that is much more expansive than simply the absence of disease, I argue in Chapter 2 for an analytical model of causation and distribution that is applicable to both a limited focus on disease and to the broader focus on health as a cluster of basic capabilities and functionings. That is, even for those choosing to maintain the focus on disease, there are still advantages to be gained from the broader explanatory framework based on entitlements.

Re-orientating our notion of health away from disease or statistically normal functioning of biological parts and processes to the framework of basic capabilities has the potential to overcome the limitations of the currently dominant explanatory model in epidemiology. Conflating our general concern for health with the concept of disease has created much confusion in our understanding of the variety of concerns we group under the heading of health as well as for how and what we identify as the causes, consequences and distribution patterns of health.

The field of epidemiology, which is the informational engine of public health programmes and clinical medicine, identifies the causes, distribution and effective treatments of diseases or impairments in individuals. Yet, contrary to the impression given by the prodigious amounts of health research being published in academic and popular press, a divisive debate is taking place among epidemiologists. It concerns whether the determinants of disease can only include individual-level 'biomedical' factors such as genetic endowment, exposures to physical substances and individual behaviours or whether supra-individual factors such as social processes that have influence through psychobiological pathways and the conditions that set up the proximate factors can also be legitimate determinants. Part of the tumult is described as disagreements about the hierarchy of evidence (Kelly et al., 2010). As Mike Kelly points out, there are two levels of explanatory systems that are important when looking at the health of populations, one at the individual level and one at the population level (Kelly et al., 2010). The evidence at the population level seems to be less 'hard' than at the individual level. I would argue that at the heart of the debate is the conflict over whether epidemiology should move forward as a natural science seeking to objectively explain natural phenomena or whether it is an instrumental and social science with a social mission (Krieger, 1994; Susser and Susser, 1996a, 1996b; Rothman et al., 1998; Marmot, 2006; Venkatapuram and Marmot, 2009).

Social epidemiology, or social determinants of health research is directly questioning the completeness of the dominant model which examines only discrete, proximate exposures and short causal chains. Social epidemiologists highlight the broader interactive and iterative processes between the individual and the environment over the life course. And the substantive amount of insightful findings means that a new epidemiological model of causation and distribution is needed that can capture both the biomedical causal factors as well as the social causes, from the local to the global, over the entire life course (Susser, 1994a, 1994b; Susser and Susser, 1996a, 1996b; Marmot, 2005, 2006).

Epidemiologists and others may learn valuable lessons by comparing what a traditional biomedical analysis of the causation and distribution of starvation would produce versus using Drèze and Sen's entitlement analysis. Geoffrey Rose made the point that we should recognize the difference between determinants of disease in individuals and incidence rates in different populations. Explanations of individual level phenomenon such as starvation due to the lack of food are different from explanations of starvation at the population level and its social distribution. That is, individuals starving from the lack of food aggregated together do not provide a sufficient explanation for the occurrence of starvation in a population, the persistence of famine starvation over generations, the avoidance of famines in other populations, or allow the recognition of asymmetrical distribution of malnutrition in a population. Drèze and Sen saw this gap between individual and group level analysis in the fact starvation mortality was avoided even where there was no food available locally, and starvation mortality occurred even where food was available locally.

The population level analysis has to be informed by the individual level analysis, and can subsume the individual level analysis. But the individual level analysis cannot provide insight beyond the individual level. For this reason, a population level analytical framework can serve better as a general theory of the epidemiology. The challenge facing modern epidemiology is to understand the phenomenon at the individual and population level, and explicate the causal pathways between the population and individual levels. The entitlement analysis successfully shows how to do this regarding impairments and mortality related to acute and endemic malnutrition. I am arguing that it can do even more as it can help analyse all causes of impairments and mortality and their social distribution; the entitlement analysis is essentially the analysis of the capability to be adequately nourished, and it can be generalized to evaluate the capability to be healthy more broadly.

Part II

In Part II there is a shift to developing an argument for a moral entitlement to a CH in line with the CA developed by Sen and Nussbaum (Sen, 1999a; Nussbaum, 2006). In Chapter 3, I review the basic concepts in the CA, discuss some of the major differences between Sen and Nussbaum, and point out some issues at the frontier of the theory. In Chapter 4, the ethical argument for the CH is presented. At the risk of repeating much of what I presented above, it is argued that every human being has a moral entitlement to the social bases of a sufficient and equitable CH because of its intrinsic value in constituting human dignity as well as its instrumental value for conceiving, pursuing and revising ('pursuing') one's own life plans within contemporary global society. The CH is grounded in the fundamental values of liberty and equality. The argument makes use of both the Senian capability 'analytical device' as well as Nussbaum's normative argument for pre-political entitlements to basic capabilities (Nussbaum, 2000b; Robeyns, 2005a). As such, the CH argument presented here is a Sen-Nussbaum 'hybrid' argument.

The CH argument is, as I stated earlier, also indebted to the work of Lennart Nordenfelt (Nordenfelt, 1987; Nordenfelt et al., 2001). His trenchant critique of the biostatistical theory and other theories of health as well as his argument for health as an ability to achieve vital goals makes it possible and plausible to see health as a capability particularly, a cluster of capabilities. As such, Nordenfelt's work helps bridge capability theory and the longstanding discussions in the philosophy of health, biology and medicine. At the end of the section, I also briefly consider how it is possible to reach the idea of a right to CH through Francis Kamm's arguments on the 'goods of life'.

Part III

As part of the dialectical reasoning about the entitlement to the CH, the discussion in Part III confronts the argument with how other ethical approaches deal with health claims. The discussion in Chapter 5 focuses in particular on the health equity criteria put forward by Margaret Whitehead, the health and human rights paradigm as well as welfare and resource theories of distributive justice including a recent luck egalitarian argument. Indeed, one can list a large number of other approaches to social justice such as libertarianism, feminism, communitarianism, republicanism, multiculturalism and so forth. My reason for focusing on the CA and these five alternatives is that they are the dominant approaches in real-world health policy or in the academic deliberations about distributive justice. Chapter 6 focuses on how the CA is faced with the challenge of the status of groups within the theory. The notion of population health, or the implicit understanding in social epidemiology and in health sociology that populations have emergent properties, and that they are not just the aggregation of individuals, presents a challenge to the CA which espouses ethical individualism. Should groups be given ethical status? Or, is group level analysis primarily to provide information about the individual members within the groups?

Chapter 7 discusses the implications of a species-wide conception of health and the related moral claims for discussions about cosmopolitanism and global justice. I argue that any theory of social justice which gives attention to health, as every theory of justice must do, will have to rely on a conception of health as capability, which is a species wide ethical idea and source of moral claims. As a result, using such a conception of health explodes out any theory of social justice into one that is at least minimally cosmopolitan. Any theory of justice will have to recognize the moral claims of every human being for their CH wherever we find them.

Finally, while the driving motivation behind formulating the argument for a moral entitlement to the CH has been that the CA has something significant to contribute to our ethical reasoning on health and justice, the argument in turn produces some suggestions for advocates of the many versions of the CA to consider. As I said earlier, focusing on the capability to be healthy of people can tell us much about our theories and principles of social justice. So the concluding chapter of the book presents some of those points CA advocates might consider as they continue to develop the CA. It reviews what are seen to be the main contributions of this book and also looks forward to some of the next questions.

The scope and limitations of this argument

Every book and every argument has its limitations. Each of the seven chapters could easily be expanded into a book, but the guiding aim of the present project is to illustrate how the idea of a human right or a moral right to health can be made coherent and justifiable. Almost immediately since it was articulated in international human rights law, and even after enormous recent scholarship, the right to health is dismissed as incoherent; the most frequent move is to interpret it as a right to healthcare.

This book aims to show how a right to health can be a coherent concept grounded in the foundational values of justice. The argument also aims to show how a capability to be healthy can be meaningfully articulated within the CA and be supported by the sciences. It also aims to show how the CA handles health issues better than alternative ethical and technical approaches. Striving to achieve these goals required diving deep into some foundational concepts in the health sciences, in social sciences and in ethics. This has also meant being less attentive to a number of relevant disciplines, asking ambitiously expansive questions, and becoming exposed to the benefits and pitfalls of inter-disciplinary research. Indeed, the CA is amenable and promotes such an effort. It has been described as 'post-disciplinary' as it can potentially bring together a variety of disciplines cutting across empirical and normative analysis (Robeyns, 2002). And that is shown to be true here.

Others also recognize that reasoning about health and morality at the level of societies or populations requires multi-disciplinary thinking; that the biological and medical sciences have to be brought together with social sciences and ethics (Anand et al., 2006; Asada, 2007). In any case, the value of putting forward the basic architecture of a capability to be healthy within a prescribed word limit is seen to be worth paying the price of giving less consideration to a range of other issues. The limitations are identified throughout the discussion. Making the capability to be healthy central to the theory and realization of social justice is a long-term project, and this book serves as the first instalment.

Two final thoughts

I end this already lengthy introduction with two thoughts. The intuitive appeal to me personally of the CA lies in its grounding in the lives of human beings wherever they are in the world, particularly those individuals who suffer the most deprivations. It has immediate relevance to realizing justice in the world. Over fifteen years ago, it also had intuitive appeal in light of first-hand experience addressing the spread of HIV/AIDS which showed that it is not healthcare or technology that was most important when saving lives. Rather, successful prevention and care strategies required engendering people's control over their own body and behaviour over the lifespan as well as changing the surrounding social conditions. The concept of capabilities nicely captured the internal and external factors that need to be addressed in order for people to avoid fatal infections over the life course.

Nevertheless, there was a remarkable disconnect between the CA and mainstream academic discussions in political philosophy on social justice. Sen, Nussbaum and their arguments were thought to be peripheral to the most interesting and central debates in social justice philosophy. Bringing up the spread of HIV/AIDS or the health of poor women in poor countries in political philosophy seminars usually resulted in sniggers or patronizing dismissals. Things have changed dramatically. Addressing global inequality and the persistence of poor health of the worst-off in the world are now seen to be very interesting and novel philosophical problems. And it is the capabilities approach that is the most entrenched in those concerns.

Furthermore, in his final writings John Rawls makes a great effort to explain how Sen's capabilities are reflected in his theory. In fact, Rawls writes, 'His [Sen's] idea is essential because it is needed to explain the propriety of the use of primary goods' (Rawls, 1999, p. 13). If my personal affinity for the CA nor the fact that it is closest to the issues of human deprivations do not convince, perhaps that the most renowned modern philosopher of social justice makes such an effort to highlight the importance of the idea of capabilities will behove academic philosophers to give the CA a bit more concerted attention.

Lastly, a passage written by Thomas Pogge I read over ten years ago has stayed with me. He writes that academic philosophers find speaking truth to power not intellectually exciting so they tend to talk to each other and focus on the intra-academic gaps (Pogge, 2001, p. 3). Recalling this passage helps me keep perspective as I sit through onerous seminars, plough through hundreds of pages of sometimes dense and esoteric scholarship, or meet philosophers who seem primarily interested in the possible novel aspects of human deprivations. Pogge's words help me remember that just because philosophers do not find some ideas or issues philosophically interesting does not meant that they are not an obvious and important part of social justice.

This book is meant to forge a path somewhere in between polemics and intellectual novelty. It seeks to help concerned individuals speak

truth to power about the injustice in the causation, persistence, distribution, levels and differential experience of impairments and mortality
of human beings within and across modern societies. The book also
aims to make some contributions to the academic debates on health
and social justice by advancing an argument for a right to the capability to be healthy. If it is even modestly successful in achieving these
two aims, I will be immensely satisfied.

Part I

1

Health as Capability

The concepts of health and disease as well as related ideas such as illness, disability, impairment and so forth have profound importance in modern societies. A range of rights and obligations, often of great material significance and life-or-death consequence, flow from how these concepts are defined. Even at the international level, the concepts of health and disease are frequently used to evaluate societies or compel global action. The background or tacit understanding in the medical professions is that a person is healthy if she has no disease. And such a notion of disease is broad in that it includes infectious disease, chronic disease, injuries, poisonings, growth disorders, functional impairments and so on; all the conditions that are seen to be deviation from 'normal' or 'natural' functioning and the life course of a human being. And in public health or health policy-making, the aim is often to 'contain and control' diseases that lead to impairments and mortality. In doing this, such policies are seen to be improving or protecting health. The concept of disease, then, plays a crucial role in our conception of health.

The following discussion seeks to break the mutuality between disease and health, and also undermine some related views. Such views include seeing health 'needs' as largely requirements for healthcare goods and services or seeing the scope of health policy as being limited to healthcare policy, which, in the view of some, should be more accurately called 'sickness care policy'. The following discussion on the scientific or medical understanding of health and disease is also aimed to express scepticism about measuring health as time lived without disease as many health economists do, and about conceptions of health in social justice literature as 'normal range of species typical functioning'.

For anyone seeking to advance ethical or justice claims related to health or health-related goods, or even for arguments for how individuals should treat or relate to each other with respect to health, it is crucial to come to grips with the prevailing notion of health as well as to have a clear grasp of the health-related concepts that are being deployed in one's own argument. Without a solid understanding of the dominant view of health, what is wrong with it, why it perseveres, and how the health concepts we are using stand in comparison, the claims we personally advocate could become vulnerable. Blindly relying on existing concepts of health and disease could wholly undermine our reasoning if the underlying concept is shown to be incoherent. Such vulnerability and incoherence is indeed evident in much of the health and human rights, health equity, or health and social justice literature.

There is also a growing body of sophisticated analysis concerning whether we should be worried about the causes, consequences or inequalities of health, or if we should be focused on inequalities of health across individuals or groups. But, it becomes clear quite quickly upon closer examination that even there the concept of health is used without much scrutiny. As Alan Cribb rightly describes it, health often seems to be 'merely a useful compound label' for a variety of things (Cribb, 2001, p. 22).

Though this chapter is not meant to be a historical project, the first section discusses some main points from the large body of literature that has developed critically evaluating the dominant view of health as the absence of disease. Such an overview is aimed to bring anyone interested in health justice up to speed in the philosophy of health and medicine debates. This is not the place for a comprehensive review as that would be a diversion from the primary goal of putting forward a concept of health as a capability. I aim broadly to lay out the theory underlying the prevailing view of health and its major criticisms, contribute some of my own criticisms, and lastly, present and extend an alternative theory of health.

The theory of health I am advancing rejects the plausibility and pursuit of a value-free and scientific notion of health, or one that is wholly centred on the concept of disease. Instead, I argue for a conception of health as a person's ability to achieve or exercise a cluster of basic human activities. These activities are in turn specified through reasoning about what constitutes a minimal conception of a life with equal human dignity in the modern world. I arrive at this conception by modifying Lennart Nordenfelt's theory of health, which defines health as the ability to achieve vital goals (Nordenfelt, 1987; Nordenfelt et al., 2001). I extend rather than wholly graft Nordenfelt's argument into my project because it suffers from what I consider to be two significant drawbacks.

While Nordenfelt develops a plausible and coherent account of human health as the ability to achieve set of vital goals, he makes vital goals relative to each community and significantly dependent on individual preferences. By doing so, he comes up against problems with both socially relative concepts of health and subjectively defined well-being. Though there is important value in a community determining what constitutes vital goals for its members, Nordenfelt's theory may under-recognize how social norms can actually impede the abilities of some individuals to achieve vital goals, or how certain valuable human functionings are not valued by the social norms of certain societies (e.g. female literacy, sexuality, or mobility). And, regarding preferences, even if a theory of informed preferences was deployed to counteract problems like expensive tastes or adaptive preferences, the central role given to preferences or subjective well-being in defining the health of a person is problematic. It is difficult if not impossible to compare the subjective experience of individuals. There needs to be an external viewpoint in addition to a person's subjective viewpoint in determining whether a person is healthy or to what extent they are healthy.

Moreover, even when an individual's preferences and the society's social norms coincide, they both can evidence parochialism that undermines the achievement of vital human goals of outsiders and future generations. Where sparse material conditions of some communities lead to community norms endorsing fewer vital goals or lower thresholds of vital goals, Nordenfelt's definition – as it stands now – would still consider that to be healthy. Overcoming both the drawbacks of subjective preferences and 'bounded' social norms and conditions in defining vital goals or health requires objective reasoning across human communities and individuals.

The theory of health proposed here replaces Nordenfelt's empty set of preferences and society-relative vital goals with a human species-wide conception of basic vital goals, or 'central human capabilities and functionings'. As a result, the health of an individual should be understood as the ability to achieve a basic cluster of beings and doings – having the capability to achieve a set of inter-related capabilities and functionings. Importantly, health is not defined by assessing the achievements of certain basic functionings or outcomes but by assessing the capability to achieve certain capabilities and functionings. But in some cases the only way to measure capabilities may be to measure actual achievements. Furthermore, by making health a 'meta' or overarching capability of exercising a cluster of capabilities, we are able to bridge the biomedical focus on the presence or absence of disease and its everyday social usage which usually describes an individual's subjective well-being and abilities to function in the world. That is to say, one of the capabilities within a cluster of health capabilities is the capability of avoiding disease, and it is one among a range of other capabilities related to how the individual is feeling and doing things in the world.

The meta-capability concept also bridges philosophy of health and medicine debates with the debates on the capabilities approach and indeed, debates on social justice more generally. Theories of justice which seek to address health issues will now have a bridge to philosophy of health debates through the concept of health as a capability rather than simply deferring to prevailing notions or gliding superficially over the debates. Furthermore, I will argue that by integrating Nordenfelt's theory with a theory of basic human capabilities such as that of Martha Nussbaum, some of the criticisms against Nordenfelt's theory fall away. So to begin, first, I shall review the theory of health as the absence of disease, then Nordenfelt's theory, and then, present my argument for conceiving health as the capability to achieve a basic set of capabilities and functionings.

Biostatistical theory of health (BST)

Starting in the early1960s contentious debates ensued in the United States and the United Kingdom over the scientific objectivity of the concept of disease and related concepts such as health, illness, malady and disability (Szasz, 1960; Marmor, 1972; Stoller et al., 1973; Blaxter, 2010). The debates centred on a position seen to be extreme and polemical – that 'disease' is simply a socially constructed category reflecting socially disvalued conditions or behaviours. These debates were initially within the field of psychiatry concerned with the definition of mental illness, but they quickly broadened out to all of medicine or healthcare. As a direct response to the debates Christopher Boorse published a series of four articles in the late 1970s with the aim of establishing a scientific and value-free definition of health and illness (Boorse, 1975, 1976a, 1976b, 1977).

Boorse's ambitious aim was to create a theory of health as well as a theory of medicine, since the aim of medical practice is generally understood to be to address the health needs of human beings. He assumed, like so many others still do, that clinical medicine/healthcare and human health are mutually encompassing ideas. If the concept of health is defined, then the scope and purpose of medicine becomes defined; if the scope of medicine is defined, then health becomes defined, a supposedly perfect mutuality.

While the notion of health as the absence of disease preceded Boorse, during the three decades following its initial presentation, Boorse's theory has indeed become standard in medical teaching and practice. At the same time, it has provoked tremendous criticism and often serves as the referent background theory to much of the philosophy of health and medicine literature. Boorse's argument for 'theoretical health' presented in its amended 1997 form contains the following four components:

The *reference class* is a natural class of organisms of uniform functional design; specifically, an age group of a sex of a species.

A *normal function* of a part or process within members of the reference class is a statistically typical contribution by it to their individual survival and reproduction.

A *disease* is a type of internal state which is either an impairment of normal functional ability, i.e. a reduction of one or more functional abilities below typical efficiency, *or a limitation on the functional ability caused by environmental agents.* [emphasis mine]

Health is the absence of disease. (Boorse, 1997, pp. 7–8)

It may be helpful to recapitulate and interpret the four points in reverse, starting from the conclusion. A living thing is healthy if it is not diseased. To be diseased means that somewhere in the inter-related and organized physiological structure, a biological part or process is 'functionally reduced' to a level 'below' the normal distribution of such values (typical efficiency) in similar individuals or limited by environmental agents. Normal functioning refers only to the statistically typical contributions parts and processes make to the individual's survival and reproduction. And, an individual's functioning is compared to those of a reference class made up of other individuals of the same sex and age of the same species. The three premises and conclusion of the theory have often been summarized as health being the *absence of disease* or health as *species typical functioning*.

The basic underlying idea that Boorse is advancing is that human biological and mental functioning is geared towards or 'designed for' individual survival and reproduction. And the biological functionings of parts or processes that are not causally related to survival and reproduction are excluded from the domain of health. As a result, a physical deformity, even though it may be atypical, if it does not directly affect survival or reproduction is not categorized as disease. And if it is not a disease it does not relate to health. Moreover, instead of using the standard of ideal values or even population average values, the statistically normal distribution model makes use of a range of values that occur most frequently across a reference class or population of human beings.

The link between statistically normal and what occurs most frequently is important to recognize because not only does it acknowledge variation in functioning among the human species, it is also unable to say if someone is less or more healthy within the range of normal or typical functioning. For example, the most frequently occurring values of a functioning may not be the most efficient contribution to survival. Think of the most frequently occurring resting heart rate for a group of thirty-year-old men versus that of a sub-group of thirty-year-old male athletes. Even though the heart and other body parts of these athletes may be making a more efficient contribution to survival, the idea of frequency is only about how often something occurs. To be healthy means that the measurement values of functionings of parts and processes are not rare or atypical, and fall somewhere within the most often occurring values in an age–sex reference class.

For those unfamiliar with statistics, the graph on the next page may be helpful to understand the concept of statistical normal distribution that Boorse is using. Imagine that the graph represents the measurements of a biological part's functioning in a reference class of individuals. The different bars in the histogram represent the frequency of different values occurring in the reference class. The average value or mean is 3.8, and one standard deviation is 4.3. This means that 68.2 per cent of the values fall somewhere between 3.8 ± 4.3, and 95.4 per cent of values fall between 3.8 ± 8.6. Individuals whose 'test results' show a measurement value below -4.8 or above 12.4 would be abnormal. Boorse never actually identifies a threshold for disease.

However, if we are to follow through on the use of the statistical normal distribution cure, health would be the most frequent 95.4 per cent or 'normal range' of values, and the remaining values in the tails

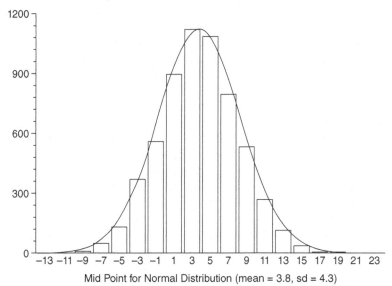

Histogram for Normal Distribution (mean = 3.8, sd = 4.3)

Mid Point for Normal Distribution (mean = 3.8, sd = 4.3)

would be disease. But Boorse thinks that people in the 'below' tail would have disease or show pathology while those on the 'above' tail may have 'positive health'. But he seems to be conflating two distinct exercises here. One is assessing simply if and at what level the organ is functioning, and the other, how well it is functioning. If it is only the first, we should classify both tails as disease, not just the 'below' tail. A heart beating too slowly and one that is beating too fast are both likely to interfere with survival and reproduction. But if we are taking measurements of functional efficiency, then the distribution is of how well the part or process is working, making the more efficient tail more acceptable as 'positive health'. But without a specific efficiency test, we are only able to plot the values of measurements and identify both tails.

In any case, Boorse also put forward a theory of illness in order to capture the social values aspects of disease and health. Recognizing the discontinuities between his objective definition and the social usage of the terms, he proposed a secondary theory of illness. He suggested the use of the term 'illness' in medical practice to identify the sub-class of diseases to which a society attaches normative judgements.

One of the more provocative aspects of Boorse's theory is that he claims that mental disease can also be defined similarly through the tabulation of the normal distribution of mental functionings across human beings. What is most common or frequent in mental function-ing across a reference class of human beings becomes the standard for what is healthy. Indeed, Boorse developed his theory initially in order to clarify psychiatric issues, but it is controversial because, unlike biological functioning, it appears easier to question the assertion that what occurs most frequently in mental functioning among a group of human beings should be viewed as what is healthy. It is perhaps in relation to mental functioning that the tension becomes clear between objectively describing health as the most frequently occurring functioning versus the idea of health as describing an ideal or excellence in human functioning.

Boorse's theory of disease, health and illness has profoundly shaped the parameters of the debates in the philosophy of health and medicine since the 1970s. The idea of health as being a range of species typical functioning and a threshold (i.e. the lower tail) has also been used in political philosophy (Daniels, 1985; Rawls, 1993, pp. 182–185). Despite the number and range of criticisms accumulating for many years, Boorse attempted a rebuttal only in 1997 (Boorse, 1997). Since then, he has also presented commentaries on the some of the leading alternative theories (Boorse, 2002, 2004). In the 1997 rebuttal Boorse bundles all the numerous critiques into three general categories including technical objections, objections from biology and objections from medicine. I focus here on three criticisms related to the baseline of functionings and role of the environment, the notion of pathology, and biological purpose as they highlight the weaknesses that I find particularly troublesome.

The baseline and the environment

To start with the first criticism, referring back to his four-point formulation as stated in 1997, Boorse argues that a disease is either a reduction below typical efficiency or a limitation of functioning caused by environmental factors. The first type of reduction entails a comparison of functioning between individuals and their reference class. The second type of limitation refers to the decrease in functionings of an entire population. He added the second clause in 1997 in order to accommodate for environmental catastrophes where the entire population is affected; where the entire population distribution curve shifts. What Boorse initially thought of as a fixed baseline of species-typical functioning he now recognizes can move, such as when the entire population is affected by a common factor. Without adding such a clause, reduced health functionings in an individual would be classified as healthy because the rest of the population would also have reduced functionings. This problem arises as a direct consequence of health being defined as the most frequent or common occurrence, rather than reflecting another principle such as the best, ideal or excellence of functioning of a human being.

This amendment, however, does not solve Boorse's problem regarding the influence of the environment on the entire reference class or entire population. Industrial accidents like Chernobyl or Union Carbide can indeed affect so many people that one would need a way to escape defining health wholly as the most frequently occurring values in a population. However, this amendment is only useful if one thinks that the baseline before the environmental event was somehow objective or natural. And the clause depends on recognizing changes in the distribution of values before and after a visible or sudden environmental event with exposure to material 'agents'. Let me address the latter point first. Where no such discrete event occurs, or something like blanket air pollution is not visible, the majority of the population may still be exhibiting reduced functionings due to less patently obvious factors or agents.

For example, let us assume that we did not know that smoking causes lung cancer and other impairments. If every member of a population smokes, and it has always been so, we would not be able to tell that the people were experiencing reduced lung functioning. And, if we suspected that the lung functioning was reduced, we would not be able to recognize why because there would not be a comparison group which does not smoke. So, if we go by frequency, reduced lung functioning looks like the natural human condition and, if we did think that lung functioning could be better, we would probably end up looking for genetic differences between individuals as the cause.

Now consider the former point about the baseline. When we do find that smoking causes reduced lung functioning, under Boorse's theory, the level of smoking in the population will determine what we consider to be normal lung functioning. There is no environmental limitation, as Boorse imagines, related to smoking, so what is most frequent functioning would still continue to be what is healthy. If we use another cause of disease, such as consumption of alcohol, salt or fat, we still have the same problem.

The research from social epidemiology shows that distribution of life expectancy and health functionings across the entire population are determined by social processes and institutions (Marmot and Wilkinson, 1999; Berkman and Kawachi, 2000). How people relate to each other, entrenched social norms, or average social practices may be holding back the entire distribution curve from where it could otherwise be. What is considered to be a healthy value now because it is within the most frequently occurring range could move to the disease part of the distribution if the social arrangements were different. The consequence of this is that the baseline of typical functioning of a population is socially determined; it is not a natural baseline. The measurements can be natural facts, but the causes of the natural facts do not originate in nature. Broad social determinants influence the baseline of health functionings, and this is a large part of what makes up the differences in health achievements across national populations.

This is an important contrast with the environmental agents scenario. The knowledge that an entire distribution of values could be shifted through social policies towards where the biological parts make more or less efficient contribution to survival and reproduction undermines the notion of the most frequently occurring values as being objectively healthy. Rather than comparing a distribution with the distribution before a sudden or visible event affecting the entire population, the more plausible comparison is the current distribution with where it could *potentially* shift to through supportive social policies. One way to recognize the possibility of shifting the entire distribution curve is to compare it with another societal population (Rose, 1985). Comparison with another population which survives longer would show that it is biologically possible for an entire population to achieve better functionings, and that the differences are likely to be in the social differences between the two populations.

Boorse could respond that the reference class includes all relevant members of the human species, so there is no second population to identify a possibly better distribution of functionings; all the values would be present in the distribution. This response, however, still does not do away with the point that even a human species-wide reference class could be functioning at a reduced level in comparison to a possible, better distribution that could be achieved through changing the social determinants of biological functionings. To put it simply, the baseline of the normal distribution of biological functioning in a population is not purely a natural phenomenon, or affected wholly only by material environmental agents. Social factors within human populations, whether within societies, or within a reference class across the human species, can shift the entire distribution curve. This makes Boorse's line demarcating disease and health within reference classes contingent on current social arrangements.

Perhaps an example will help. The life expectancy of fruit flies or zebras has not changed over the last century. The most frequent functionings in a population of fruit flies or zebra could be a considered a natural baseline. But human life expectancy has been constantly lengthening because we have been influencing human behaviours and their external and physical conditions. We have also been changing their biology through such things as vaccinations. The fact that biological functionings are profoundly determined by social arrangements undermines Boorse's assertion that the most frequently occurring range of values in a human population is a value-free, scientific account of health.

One possible solution for Boorse is to amend his definition to include a stipulation that disease is functioning limited by environmental factors as well as social factors. This move would try to restore the natural baseline away from the influence of both environmental and social influences. But such a move seems profoundly to misunderstand the human animal. Human beings are and will probably continue to be born from and among other human beings. And the social context of human beings is what has contributed to increasing life expectancy and control of impairments. The sociability of the human animal, like other primates, is an intrinsic part of its characteristics and also determines its physiological functionings and longevity. The social aspects of human beings are literally written on the bodies of human beings. Presenting a natural baseline of functionings that discounts the impact of social factors misunderstands the human animal by trying to exclude the influence of its sociability on its physiological functioning. While Boorse may be right in trying to capture the difference between organic matter and a living organism, he is unwilling to distinguish between the striving of any living thing and that of human beings. Because human beings can and do change the baseline of health functionings through social action, the baseline and consequent thresholds of disease and health are not natural. No other living organisms can intentionally change their baseline of functionings. The fact that human beings can is what makes it impossible to be value neutral about the baseline, and what makes health a normative concept.

Other environment objections

Aside from the issue that the baseline of human functioning is not wholly naturally determined, Boorse's theory is still open to other environment related criticisms. First, it conceives of human beings as functioning at one constant level. For the BST to make sense, one has to imagine a human body of either sex at a particular age working like a machine that functions at a constant rate. Critics of the BST have pointed out that humans carry out various activities in different environments, and that biological functionings are dynamic, making possible short-term adaptations to changing conditions in the environment. As the temperature becomes hotter, colder, or as the altitude increases, the body's physiological processes adapt in order to reach some level of homeostasis. The BST does not account for the body's ability to alter functionings in order to adapt to changes in the environment. The model just compares what one body part or process is doing in comparison to the rest of the reference class. Some of the adaptive processes can be short term, such as perspiration, and others can be long term, such as changes in metabolism. By not taking into account the ability of the body to adapt, the BST will misclassify individuals as being diseased, when they are actually adapting to their immediate environment in order to survive. However, in order to be fair, this misclassification of individuals as being diseased while they are only adapting will happen on the margins; people who are on the edges of the normal distributions and move into certain environments results in the values falling outside the normal distribution. But can a theory of health that seeks to be scientific and objective afford to be so fuzzy on the edges?

A slightly different adaptation criticism is that the BST ignores what the individual is actually doing and thus will misclassify individuals as diseased when they are undertaking different kinds of activities that alter their biological functionings. Unlike in the previous examples where the body adapts to changes in the environment, here, a person pursuing an activity such as running a sprint or marathon would be identified as exhibiting abnormal functioning relative to the reference class. Assuming that her entire reference class is also not running a sprint or marathon, during the period when the body is fully exerting itself, the BST would classify her as diseased because her measurements of particular biological parts or processes would probably fall outside the normal distribution range of her reference-class. But, nevertheless, we would think it odd to consider the person diseased or unhealthy.

The changes in functionings because of having to adapt to changing environments or when undertaking various activities reveals the necessity to take into account the interaction between the individual and the environment. Yet, the BST holds constant both the activity and the environment. In order not to classify these individuals as diseased, it would have to incorporate all adaptations in all environments as well as the range of functionings during all activities as being within the normal range. But this would mean the BST would lose substantial analytical power in being able to differentiate between normal and abnormal. The theory would not be able to differentiate between a person who is running a marathon from a person who is just short of experiencing hypothermia or a person who is sleeping. By including all the values related to all activities and adaptations, it would become too all encompassing to offer any meaningful distinctions.

Boorse's reply is that he had initially recognized these two types of environmental challenges but assumed that averaging across a large reference class would take care of these variations. That is, if the measurements of a large enough group is used, then the measurements of a person when she is resting, when she is in a cold environment, or when she is running a marathon would all fall under the normal distribution. But then, it is unclear how one tells the difference between the biological functioning of someone who is running a marathon and someone who is functioning abnormally. If these environmental and adaptation issues do indeed persist then, according to Boorse, the theory only requires adding in the stipulation 'in a statistically normal environment'. Putting in the stipulation of a standard environment means the range of normal values of a functioning is linked to a particular standard environment; as the standard environmental conditions change, the range of normal functioning values also moves with it. Thus, a person living at high altitudes would be compared with others living at high altitudes in contrast to being compared to the entire reference class. This would also presumably apply to all the different types of activities individuals could carry out in a particular environment. One compares an individual with a reference class of individuals in a similar environment carrying out the same or similar activities.

While this may satisfy Boorse, standardizing the environment has significant additional implications that he either is unaware of or ignores. When the biological functioning of a reference class is standardized to a particular environment, it means that it is also localized to a particular geographical location in the world. The consequence is that the definitions of disease and health are no longer a human species-wide conception but become geographically relative or specific to a sub-group of human species. This could be a plausible option if human beings were animals that were only reactive agents living in nature. That is to say, in evolutionary theory, animals adapt to their geographic environments, and the most common resultant features can be considered healthy; the most common features contribute to their reproduction and survival. But because human beings are able to transform their surrounding environments, for better or worse, which in turn affect their biological and mental functioning, the distribution of their functionings do not have the same 'naturalness' as feather

colours or beak shapes. Categorizing adaptations in biological functionings as normal even though they were self-induced by some level
of human influence on the physical and social environment introduces
values into the definition of health.

For example, the increasing average height of many national populations is often attributed to changes in diet and nutrition of the most
recent generations. The ability of human beings to alter directly or
indirectly their own biological functions counters the idea that biological functioning is naturally designed for survival and reproduction, and
their adaptations are directed to reaching those goals. Moreover, referring again to Rose, the evaluation of the biological functionings of
human populations would be incomplete without comparing them to
other human population groups (Rose, 1985). So, in fact, we do not
always want to standardize an environment to a given population, we
want to compare populations making the environment the variable
factor. We often want to change the environment to make the entire
population function better or more healthily. Lastly, the 'statistically
normal environment' stipulation really produces the biggest problem
where the statistically normal environments and political borders
overlap. That would mean that whatever the prevailing distributions of
health functionings are in a country or continent, those range of functionings would be considered healthy. The overlap of standard environment with social groups, particularly politically defined groups, would
lead to Boorse's BST losing much of its value-neutral pretensions.

Defence mechanisms as healthy

A second conceptual flaw of the BST is that it categorizes processes
the body initiates to ward off disease as being healthy (Nordenfelt
et al., 2001, p. 15). Because biological processes to fight disease occur
frequently in most human beings, the processes do not fall outside the
normal distribution of functionings. For example, when an infectious
organism enters the body, the immune system marshals a variety of
processes geared towards fighting off the infection. We would normally call the infection a disease and the body's process of fighting it
a period of illness. Yet, from the perspective of the BST, all of these
functionings occur in a statistically normal way and contribute to the
goal of survival and reproduction of the organism. Thus, the BST
cannot recognize the body's response to an infection as being not in
health. Boorse's response to this is that indeed, such immune responses
are normal (Boorse, 1997).

However, he argues that the disease lies in the injury at the point of entry of the infection, and any consequent death of cells. The death or decrease in functioning of cells consequent to infection defines disease. But if the death of a single cell can mean disease, then every human being is theoretically diseased. Surprisingly, Boorse concurs that, indeed, according to his theory every human being is likely to have a disease because every human being has a part or process that is not like 95.4 per cent of their reference class. Yet, this is supposedly not a theoretical deficiency. Everybody can be theoretically diseased, but only some diseases are considered illnesses requiring a social response through clinical medicine. So if we are to adhere to Boorse's theory, a person with a few dead skin cells may not have an illness but because they have a disease, they also cannot be thought of as healthy. That is to say, under Boorse's theory one dead skin cell would categorize a person as unhealthy but not as being ill.

Biological purpose

A third critique of the BST relates to how it deals with the intersection between the age reference class and the supposed biological goals of survival and reproduction. The reason Boorse includes the age reference group is because human beings obviously begin a process of physiological development starting from conception and go on to experience the degenerative aspects of ageing. At the same time as this process is occurring, Boorse identifies individual survival and reproduction as the goals of normal biological functionings. Critics have questioned the choice of survival and reproduction as the two primary biological goals as well as the possibility of conflict between them. One question to ask is what is the point of health or biological functioning in a woman who has already reproduced and is post-menopausal? From an evolutionary biology perspective, which BST clearly exhibits, the survival of post-menopausal women becomes irrelevant because they have already achieved their goal of reproduction. One way to respond to this criticism is to change the requirement from 'and' to 'or'; survival or reproduction. As a result the biological functionings in the reference class of menopausal women could still be put on a normal distribution curve. But of course, this issue could also affect men who have reproduced. Allowing the goals of survival to be separate from reproduction may have significant problems for Boorse's theory.

What then are we to make of those other situations where human beings face a choice between reproduction and survival? For human beings, survival and reproduction can sometimes be mutually exclusive goals; one impedes the other. Boorse responds that because of the ubiquity of 'parental sacrifice in reproduction', he expects the BST of health to prefer reproduction over survival (Boorse, 1997, p. 94). By which Boorse means that normal pregnancy and birth already put considerable stress on women's bodies, and if ageing or even horrible death had a reproductive function then it could not be called a disease. Boorse's understanding of functions means that the processes of a women's pregnancy and of giving birth could never be considered disease or unhealthy even if it is directly undermining her survival. Normal functioning and dying prematurely from childbirth are seen as compatible notions.

In spite of these and many other criticisms, Boorse continues to maintain that the BST still does the best job of providing a scientific and value-free conception of disease and health (Boorse, 1997, 2004). In the thirty or more years since he originally presented it, Boorse has made only one amendment to the theory regarding the influence of the environment. He seems to conclude that his critics are really more exercised about how to conceptualize health as being more than just the absence of disease than in criticizing his theoretical analysis of the disease concept itself. At the end of his 1997 rebuttal, Boorse maintains that he still has a justifiable concept of disease though he is now more open to how it can become integrated into other theories which have normative components. What is still unclear is that despite the various academic debates on the different naturalist, normative and hybrid accounts of disease or related ideas such as illness and disorder, the concept of health is largely seen as their antonym. Almost all of the theories begin with primary concepts such as disease or malady and then define its absence as being health. I would argue that it is indeed possible to speak of the health of someone despite the individual having a disease, even in Boorsean terms. Health does not have to be a yes or no evaluation, but can be assessment of various aspects of an individual. The presence or absence of disease, seen as an impairment of a biological part or process, should be seen as one aspect of a person's health.

Nordenfelt's welfare theory of health

Partly in reaction to Boorse's theory, Lennart Nordenfelt, a Swedish philosopher, developed an alternative theory of health (Nordenfelt, 1987). He also published a counter-rebuttal to Boorse's 1997 response to critics (Nordenfelt et al., 2001). Nordenfelt sees his project as being similar to that of Boorse's in that both aim to reconfigure and bring coherence to already existing health and related concepts in healthcare and in everyday language. He refers to his theory of health as a 'welfare' theory of health because, he writes, 'To characterize a human being in terms of health or illness is to describe one aspect of the "status" of this human being, what we often call his "state of well-being"' (Nordenfelt, 1987, p. 1). And he also describes it as a 'holistic' theory because rather than starting the analysis inside the body with a biological part or process, his conception of health aims to reflect the whole person, the overall quality of a person's abilities to interact with her environment to achieve her vital goals.

The starting point of Nordenfelt's analysis is the commonplace idea that we think of health when it is not there; when there is instead, pain and disability. He then chooses 'disability' as the primary concept in constructing the definition of health rather than pain because he reasons that even though pain can be due to disability, and pain can cause one to be disabled, all causes of pain are not necessarily due to disability. For example, heartache can cause pain, but it would be misguided to say that feeling pain from heartache is not healthy. So grounding health or ill-health in the concept of pain would lead us in the wrong direction. Rejecting that starting point, and instead focusing on disability, Nordenfelt makes a linguistic move. He writes, 'Disability is a negative notion presupposing the semantic content of its positive contrary, ability. This gives the analysis of ability a primary place in my theory of health' (Nordenfelt et al., 2001, p. 67). He flips the focus from disability, which relates to the lack of health or being in 'non-health' onto the focus on the positive notion of ability, or where there is the presence of health. And then he asks, so what should a healthy person be able to do? Nordenfelt envisages human ability consisting of three parts: a human agent, their goal of action, and a supportive environment in order to create the 'real practical possibility of action' (Nordenfelt, 1987, p. 41, 1993, p. 17).

This concept of practical possibility of action is further informed by the philosophy of action-theory, a disciplinary field which assesses ideas such as human action, causality, intent, basic action and action-chains (O'Connor and Sandis, 2010). In any case, aside from the different starting points, here lies another one of the clearest differences between Boorse and Nordenfelt. The latter gives explicit and important role to the influence of the external environment on the health or functioning of the individual, while the former simply made a modest amendment regarding environmental agents affecting the entire population.

In reflecting on what abilities a healthy person should have, or what actions they should be able to perform, for ease of discussion, Nordenfelt focuses on the ultimate goals of such abilities or actions; he calls these 'vital goals' (Nordenfelt et al., 2001, p. 67). Rather than saying that an individual should be able to act in these particular ways aimed at achieving this goal, he prefers to speak directly about the goals. In reasoning about what these goals could be, he considers and then rejects both 'basic needs' and satisfying desires. Basic needs are rejected because they are instrumental to other goals, or they presuppose a concept of health. A basic need is derived from a concept of health. Desire satisfaction is also rejected because of harmful desires or low desires. Instead, he reasons that a vital goal of a person is 'a state of affairs that is such that it is a necessary condition for the person's minimal happiness in the long run' (Nordenfelt, 1987, p. 93).

The stipulation of 'in the long run' is to avoid health being centred on immediate pleasure and instead be in line with more long-term happiness or flourishing such as Aristotle's eudomonia. He rephrases the definition of vital goals as 'a state of affairs which is either a component of or otherwise necessary for the person's living a minimally decent life. This includes more than survival . . .' (Nordenfelt et al., 2001, p. 68). But Nordenfelt does not fully let go of the satisfying desires or preferences. He reckons that a person's desires will still have a role to play even in the deeper notions of Aristotelian happiness or human flourishing. So what Nordenfelt tries to do is distinguish general desires or wants from the wants of life's most important or core goals. I shall return to this issue of personal desires further below.

In formal terms, Nordenfelt's theory of health is as follows:[1]

> A is in health if, and only if, A has the ability, given standard circumstances, to realize his vital goals, i.e. the set of goals which are necessary and together sufficient for his minimal happiness. (Nordenfelt, 1987, p. 97)

It is important to recognize, for reasons which will become clearer further below, that rather than taking about abilities to act in particular ways aimed at achieving a vital goal, for reasons of rhetorical ease he speaks directly about the vital goals. He clearly does not mean to say that health is levels of achievement of vital goals. Health is the abilities to achieve vital goals. Minimal happiness or flourishing is conceptualized as the outcome-states or achieving goals, but the health of a person is her abilities to achieve vital goals. Furthermore, though health is having the ability to achieve vital goals, to be unhealthy is not reflected by the not achieving of the vital goals, but by lack of the second-order ability to acquire the first-order ability to achieve vital goals. Non-health is not the lack of achieving a goal but the lack of capability to produce the ability to achieve the goal. For example, either not being adequately nourished or not having the first-order ability to be nourished (e.g. feed oneself) is not enough to be labelled as being unhealthy. I am not healthy when I am not able to acquire or learn the ability to achieve adequate nutrition. If I am currently not well nourished but can become well nourished, learn or acquire the ability to be well nourished, I am still healthy. The point at which I extinguish my own second-order ability to do the first-order action, or some other biological event, someone else or an environmental factor destroys it, I then become ill or unhealthy. So a person who is voluntarily fasting is healthy. They become unhealthy or are not in health when they can no longer have the practical possibility of achieving adequate nutrition. It is particularly insightful of Nordenfelt to account for such a second-order ability. It recognizes that individuals move around different environments, and/or require learning time to adapt, or some individuals may choose not to achieve their vital goals. Nordenfelt offers the example of an African farmer moving to a Nordic country. She may not immediately be able to achieve her vital goals in the new environment but after a period of time, she develops her abilities to achieve her vital goals. The second-order ability is defined as:

> A has a second-order ability with regard to an action F, if and only if, A has the first-order ability to pursue a training-programme after the completion of which A will have the first-order ability to do F. (Nordenfelt, 1987, p. 148)

To summarize, Nordenfelt's account is that a person's health reflects the person's (second-order) abilities to achieve various vital goals which constitute minimal happiness for the person in the long run, given a particular environment or standard circumstances. Vital goals are not those that meet basic needs or satisfy general wants but refer to those activities that constitute the most important or foundational human projects, and make up a minimally decent human life. In his full account of health, Nordenfelt also addresses other concepts such as illness, malady and disease. It is not just an account of abilities and vital goals. I would argue that Nordenfelt has brought us far in the path towards a coherent account of health. His corpus of writings as a whole shows the inadequacy of Boorse's theory, and show great care in systematically articulating his own theory while also addressing a wide range of possible objections. Nordenfelt's methodological approach and architecture of the argument are extremely useful in conceptualizing health. But there are three weaknesses. I consider each in turn, and show how they could be overcome by integrating it with the social and political theory of human capabilities.

Empty set of vital goals

The first weakness is that Nordenfelt stops short of explicitly filling in the framework of vital goals with any content, even uncontroversial content. He explains why certain goals are vital but he does not identify the content of vital goals; what exactly are the vital goals that make a flourishing or minimally decent human life? More recently, Nordenfelt has argued that vital goals across societies will have a similar 'torso'. By that he means that across societies there will be some common body of content in the vital goals. He makes an analogy between different notions of health across present societies with different historical conceptions of health stating, 'Health has always had to do with a person's well-being and ability related to his or her internal somatic and mental conditions' (Nordenfelt, 2007, p. 31). Nevertheless, it is unclear why he stops short of articulating what is or could be this common body of vital goals. For example, even though he recognizes sheer survival as only one vital goal of human beings, he does not specify this as part of the 'torso'. This is at least one common vital goal across the human species, so should it not be specified in the theory? Nor does Nordenfelt consider whether any other vital goals can be considered necessary for minimal happiness or flourishing across the human species simply by virtue of them being embodied human animals.

In response to such an assessment Nordenfelt could reply that he has in fact given consideration to the substance of vital goals. In a discussion in *On the Nature of Health* he writes, 'Being alive is a necessary condition of being happy . . . Hence all the necessary conditions for maintenance of life must be included among every person's vital goals, for instance having food, having a sheltered home and having some economic security' (Nordenfelt, 1987, p. 91). And so, from this discussion we are supposedly capable of deducing at least a shortlist of shared universal vital goals across the human species. While this may be a possible path, Nordenfelt himself has not in fact produced a shortlist of vital goals, and so his set of vital goals is still remaining (seemingly) empty.

It is a biological necessity that all human beings must be surrounded by oxygen, frequently imbibe potable water and ingest adequate nutrition in order to keep functioning. Should not those activities be specified as part of vital goals? Surely, for any human being to have the practical possibility to achieve vital goals there must be some kind of minimal physical and social conditions? Nevertheless, there is nothing more to be found about human beings and their vital goals in Nordenfelt's theory of health other than human beings perform actions, are goal oriented, and seek minimal happiness in the long run.

Despite the empty set of vital goals Nordenfelt's theory is still valuable in many aspects. His theory expands the frame of discussions of the philosophy of health away from focusing only on disease and onto human actions, emphasizes the important role of the environment as well as grounds reasoning in the philosophy of ordinary language and action-theory. He also shows why health cannot be linked to immediate desires or basic needs. Careful semantic moves and linguistic philosophy are arguably necessary in reasoning about health because theories of health are inherently projects of reconstruction or reorganizing existing health-related concepts; a theory of health must be able to reorganize and bring coherence to existing scientific knowledge on biological functioning and impairments as well as practical knowledge used in medical care. Nordenfelt has, indeed, gone some way towards establishing a conceptual architecture for a health concept that brings more coherence to the health sciences and medical practice.

However, by leaving the vital goals empty and subject to 'standard circumstances' he appears to stop short of doing any social and political philosophy. Questions such as what goals are necessary for achieving minimal happiness in the long run and what is an adequate environment for achieving these goals are left completely open. A concept of health has to be much more publicly explicit about these vital goals, and organize social arrangements, or in Nordenfelt's terms, determine the standard environment accordingly. We want a conception of human health to help us determine an adequate environment rather than let the social and physical environment determine what constitutes health.

Standard circumstances

Nordenfelt is asserting, quite rightly, that health is not just a phenomenon internal to the body, found within the biological structure, but also reflects the direct influence of the environment whether through physical or social forces on the individual. When a person has no practical possibility to act because something or someone constrains their capacity of action, then they are disabled and impaired, and not in health. However, because of what appears to be complete capitulation to the local social circumstances in determining the content of vital goals for minimal happiness, Nordenfelt's formulation advocates social and ethical relativism. This is not a small issue in regard to health and longevity and is the second weakness in Nordenfelt's theory. While Nordenfelt may be reasoning about what a coherent understanding of health is, by defining it, he is also advocating for how health should be envisaged. Because it has normative aspects, his definition cannot be seen to be adequate for its complete cultural and ethical relativism. Nordenfelt does recognize this tension as he states that he thinks about local conditions as either being standard or as reasonable. He suggests that in different discourses about health, we will either accept standard or given circumstances and in others we will accept what are reasonable circumstances (Nordenfelt et al., 2001, p. 68). But that seems only to bolster the point that the definition of health is contextually dependent on what is considered standard or reasonable for that scenario. The concepts of standard and reasonable become pivotal but they come from outside his theory; it is not clear who or what body of reasoning will provide the criteria for standard or reasonable circumstances.

This conclusion that health could be assessed either in culturally/conextually relative circumstances or against what are considered to be reasonable circumstances is unsatisfying. A theory of health is needed precisely to organize or evaluate rights and obligations related to health where local circumstances conflict with or fall well below what are considered to be reasonable circumstances. One of the clearest illustrations of where common social practices and individual vital goals are not aligned is evinced in the high levels of endemic and acute mortality of girls and women in developing countries. Aside from biological vulnerability, the social, political and economic practices that are locally determined undermine the abilities of girls and women to achieve basic functionings around the world. In particular, poor reproductive and sexual health in girls and women because of 'standard' patriarchal cultural norms leads to millions of avoidable deaths and impairments every year (Murray and Lopez, 1996).

Beyond the particular issue of women's health, the role of social arrangements in the causation and distribution of preventable mortality and disease is profound and pervasive across all human societies. Because the standard environment, or cultural norms can conflict with the achievement of vital goals of individuals, especially of those who are socially powerless, local cultural practices should not have absolute or overwhelming determining power over the content of vital goals, and consequently in determining who can achieve them, when, where and how long. It is also important that we recognize the important influence, whether good or bad, of the social circumstances on how individuals identify and pursue their own vital goals. The choices we make depend on the choices we have. We want a conception of health to be informed by but not wholly determined by local conditions and practices.

Nordenfelt takes us far by defining health as the abilities to achieve vital goals that lead to minimal happiness or minimally decent life, but then suggests that these vital goals can either be locally determined or according to reasonable circumstances. In order for it to be a theory of health that covers the entire human species, the empty or socially relative definition of vital goals has to be replaced with at least a core, species-wide definition of vital goals. In searching for such a species-wide conception of minimal human welfare or well-being, there are a range of options. Indeed, I could endeavour to identify a conception of vital goals based on my reasoning of reasonable circumstances. However, it seems more prudent to draw on the state-of-the-art philosophical debates on human well-being. In doing so, the overlap between Nordenfelt's vital goals and the idea of basic or central human capabilities advocated by Amartya Sen and Martha Nussbaum is quite remarkable. Nordenfelt's argument quite literally connects the debates on the philosophy of health and biology and the theory of capabilities through his idea of health as the abilities to achieve vital goals. Nordenfelt's ability to achieve vital goals is analogous to capabilities. Perhaps the overlap should not be very surprising as both Nordenfelt and the CA are informed by Aristotelian reasoning on action, influence of the environment, and human flourishing (Nordenfelt and Lindahl, 1984; Nordenfelt, 1987; Nussbaum, 1987).

Nussbaum expressly goes about identifying a conception of minimum human flourishing which is similar to Nordenfelt's vital goals necessary and sufficient for happiness in the long run. Nordenfelt is aware of the capabilities approach and has commented on relevant similarities and differences with Sen's arguments (Nordenfelt, 2000, pp. 94–105; personal communication). He recognizes that his conception of health and well-being gives greater weight to subjective mental welfare and that it concerns a smaller set of capabilities than Sen's general concern with capabilities. Nordenfelt does not, however, consider Nussbaum's arguments for a set of basic capabilities. What I am championing is that the conception of health as the abilities to achieve vital goals be combined with a list of core capabilities whereby health is being capable of or having capabilities of achieving a certain cluster of capabilities and functionings. In this view health can also be seen as a second-order or overarching capability to achieve a cluster of basic capabilities and functionings. And the bases for these capabilities being species-wide, across all societies, come from their grounding in basic human liberty and equal human dignity.

Integrating Nordenfelt and Nussbaum

Similarly to Nordenfelt, Nussbaum also finds the basic needs and desire or preference satisfaction approaches lacking in reasoning about human well-being (Nussbaum and Sen, 1993; Nussbaum, 2000b). Though Nordenfelt was thinking about a person's health in relation to human flourishing and achieving vital goals, Nussbaum's project is to define the components of a human life that reflect equal human dignity. Based on both Aristotle and Marx, she conceives human dignity as being able to be and do certain things; having certain capabilities. Placing Nordenfelt's and Nussbaum's arguments side by side shows how health and abilities or capabilities and dignity are interrelated. Through a very similar method of dialectical reasoning to Nordenfelt, but asking what kind of life is worthy of human dignity – a minimally decent human life – across all societies, Nussbaum identifies that kind of life to consist of at least a threshold level of ten capabilities (Nussbaum, 2000b, 2006). Just like Nordenfelt, Nussbaum also focuses on the abilities and not the actual achievements. In contrast to Nordenfelt's reliance on ordinary language and action-theory philosophy, Nussbaum starts in the historical debates about natural law and sees certain ethical entitlements or claims implicit in the idea of human dignity (Nussbaum, 2006, p. 37). She then identifies a life worthy of human dignity to consist of ten capabilities including: (Nussbaum, 2000b , pp. 78–80)

(1) being able to live a normal length of lifespan; (2) having good health; (3) maintain bodily integrity; (4) being able to use senses, imagination and think; (5) having emotions and emotional attachments; (6) possess practical reason to form a conception of the good; (7) have social affiliations that are meaningful and respectful; (8) express concern for other species; (9) able to play; and (10) have control over one's material and political environment. (Nussbaum, 2006: pp. 76–77)

These ten capabilities, as moral entitlements emanating from a person's human dignity, become the source of political principles for liberal pluralistic society; ensuring each member achieves a threshold level of these ten central capabilities becomes a primary political goal. So, unlike Nordenfelt who capitulates to the standard environment of various human societies or even certain setting such as clinics, Nussbaum defines what the standard environment should be in light of the moral, pre-political entitlements of human beings to the capabilities of achieving some 'beings and doings'. But her conception also has room for different societies or countries to determine the vital goals. Societies can add to the list of basic capabilities, but cannot take away capabilities from the list. And, different societies will determine the threshold levels of each capability depending on their history and resources. But these thresholds cannot be set only by domestic, 'bounded' reasoning or wholly determined by locally available circumstances. A number of issues related to the conceptualization and implementation of the list remain, which I discuss further in Chapter 5.

Indeed, Nussbaum clearly considers her list of capabilities as constituting a conception of a life of minimal human dignity and not as a conception of health. But the capabilities related to longevity and health are listed first and second on her list. And, even more intriguing is a footnote discussing the health capability in *Women and Human Development*. In the footnote, Nussbaum writes that the definition of reproductive health adopted in the Section 7 of the Final Programme of Action of the 1994 Cairo Conference on Population and Development (ICPD) 'fits well with the intuitive idea of truly human functioning that guides this list' (Nussbaum, 2000b: footnote at p. 83). That is, Nussbaum appears to be saying that the definition of reproductive health as 'a state of complete physical, mental and social well-being and not merely the absence of disease or infirmity, in all matters relating to the reproductive system and to its functions and processes' fits with what she is trying to accomplish through specifying ten central human capabilities. This definition of reproductive health in turn mimics the World Health Organization's definition of health, which, it should be noted, has frequently been disparaged as being nonsensical, utopian and unfeasible.

In any case, the implication of her drawing a parallel between the ICPD/WHO's definition of health and the list of CHCs is that it is in fact possible to define health capability as being made up of all ten capabilities. And, the footnote shows that Nussbaum is aware of at least one account of health that could possibly encompass all ten CHCs. Moreover, Nussbaum's awareness that health could be conceived as being more than just the absence of disease seems to support the notion that the health capability on her list is really about the capability to avoid disease and impairments. Otherwise, she should be putting a list of capabilities within a health capability and creating a list within a list. But why does Nussbaum still use the label of health capability instead of referring to the capability to avoid disease and impairments?

Indeed, if Nussbaum's list of capabilities proves to be troublesome as constituting health, we could develop a different set of basic capabilities. One could use alternative methodologies to come up with a different set of vital goals or capabilities, and it would still accomplish our goals of creating content for Nordenfelt's vital goals. For example, Gillian Brock argues that it is plausible to achieve global consensus on basic needs that are necessary for human agency; for 'what a human being is like' (Brock, 2005). And Ingrid Robeyns has yet another method for identifying basic human capabilities (Robeyns, 2003; Robeyns, 2005b). What is important is that the idea of health as the capability to achieve a cluster of capabilities and functionings still holds. Criticizing one capability or functioning, such as the health capability on Nussbaum's list, does not undermine the argument that health should be seen as having a cluster of basic capabilities or abilities to achieve some vital goals. To undermine that argument would entail going back and objecting to Nordenfelt's reasoning about health as being able to realize goals necessary and sufficient for minimal happiness, as in a minimally flourishing, decent, non-humiliating life in the modern world.

Thomas Schramme offers one such objection to Nordenfelt's theory. He argues that the definition of vital goals is too broad (Schramme, 2007). Schramme illustrates his objection using the example of an ambitious athlete. Lily, a high jumper, has struggled for a long time to become an accomplished athlete, but has not succeeded and is not happy. Because Lily has not achieved her minimal happiness according to Nordenfelt's theory, she is not healthy. This seems odd to Schramme, especially as Lily has no disease. Moreover, Schramme also points out that by changing her goals, by becoming less ambitious, Lily could become healthy. Schramme's critique is that the inability of Lily to achieve minimal happiness because her ambitions outstripped her physical talents should not render her unhealthy. Nordenfelt replies that he views health as being on a spectrum from complete health to maximal illness, presumably death. Therefore, Lily's unhappiness from not achieving her minimal happiness moves her down on this scale away from optimum health. But she is unlikely to be ill unless her disappointment becomes debilitating. But for such a scale to work, Nordenfelt also needs to use thresholds to distinguish optimum from moderate health, and moderate health from poor or ill-health. It is unclear where or how those thresholds will be created.

Some may find that Nordenfelt is letting a person's subjective preferences, or happiness, determine health too much. Consider the opposite, a person who has a cheery disposition despite being constrained would be considered healthy, or moderately healthy. Or, a person with low ambition or low happiness thresholds would be considered healthy. While Nordenfelt understandably links vital goals to the happiness of the individual, a strong role of the subjective experiences of happiness determining health would make the conception incoherent. And it is not sufficient to say that 'happiness in the long term' will more closely resemble Aristotelian flourishing. However, if we use Nussbaum's list of capabilities as content to Nordenfelt's vital goals, including the idea of sufficient threshold, then Lily would be considered healthy. Rather than being considered unhealthy because she is unhappy due to not becoming a stellar athlete, if she is above the thresholds of basic capabilities, she would simply be an unhappy, disappointed person. She still has sufficient abilities to achieve her ten vital goals, and health does not have to include the abilities to achieve any or all goals that will produce satisfaction or mental well-being. Nussbaum's list, by its breadth and sufficiency levels, constrains the scope of vital goals from becoming total well-being. Thereby, it also constrains what is included in the conception of health. Health represents a minimal conception of human well-being.

One of the interesting things about putting Nordenfelt's theory together with Nussbaum's capabilities is the possibility for mutual exchange. For example, Nordenfelt relies on concepts such as actor/agent, action, supportive environment and ability, which reflect his grounding in action-theory. One of the novel concepts that advocates of the CA have introduced in thinking about human actions that has implications for action-theory and the related idea of freedom more generally is that people differ in their needs for supportive environments and in their conversion skills in carrying out an action or functioning. Capability theory recognizes that the diversity in how human beings are 'constructed and situated' can affect if and how well they are able to carry out any particular act. The surrounding conditions for an act cannot be taken for granted as having uniform effects on persons, or conversely, it cannot be assumed that any act requires the same external conditions for every person. So while Nordenfelt goes far in highlighting and accounting for the influence of the environment on human ability or action, the CA carries on even further by elucidating the need to account for the individual's diversity in needs as well as in their skills to convert their own endowments and their surrounding environment in carrying out intended actions. In thinking about human actions this diversity inherent to human beings has to be taken into account.

Practical implications

The present exercise aims to move the concept of health away from what is typical or the most frequent functioning of internal biological parts and processes to one which is an evaluation of a person's capability of exercising some basic functionings in the contemporary world. This obviously implies a cascade of consequences. Foremost, reconfiguring our concept of health will affect epidemiology, the science and methodology we currently use to study the causation and distribution of what we now refer to as health though it is really the study of disease and mortality. Very few people actually study the causation of health (Huppert and Baylis, 2004; Huppert et al., 2004).

Epidemiology and other health sciences would still continue to study the causes of diseases and impairments but would also need to expand to study the causation and distribution of the cluster of basic capabilities and functionings. This is something that is already being done in social exclusion studies, development economics and in health economics (Burchardt, 2004; Anand, 2005; Anand et al., 2005; Saleeby, 2007; Coast et al., 2008a). The health sciences could provide the knowledge about the biological bases of human capabilities. Furthermore, health policy will not just be confined to preventing and managing diseases but be more broadly concerned with protecting, promoting and restoring sufficient levels of capabilities of achieving functionings. It is not that surgeons will be expected to do more than surgery but rather that what is considered to be health policy or health expertise will include more than clinical services or economic analysis of healthcare.

This reconfigured conception of health will also profoundly affect how we respond to different distributions in health, the causes of the constraints on health functionings and the differential experiences or consequences of such constraints. And importantly, this ethical concept of health as the ability to achieve certain goals is a human species-wide conception and puts the health of every human being across all societies on the same plane of observation and analysis. The concept of health is defined in terms of equal dignity of human beings in the contemporary world.

If all this talk about health as achieving vital goals or cluster of capabilities and functionings seems too theoretical or fanciful, I must note that Nordenfelt's ideas and my reconfiguration of them are not radical or revolutionary. The criticism of the BST and the exhortation that we should be redirecting healthcare and health systems towards producing health rather than narrowly on preventing and managing disease has been a longstanding cause in the health sciences (Illich, 1974). Decades ago, Aaron Antonovsky even put forward a formal 'salutogenic' theoretical model of health to guide healthcare and health policy (Antonovsky, 1979). And more recently, the World Health Assembly renamed the second edition of the International Classification of Impairments, Disabilities and Handicaps as the International Classification of Functioning, Disability and Health (World Health Organization, 2001). This renaming reflects a movement that seeks to recognize health as being a spectrum from fully functioning in the world to being fully impaired, and that which explicitly recognizes that functionings or abilities are co-produced by the features of the individual and surrounding environment. Moreover, this new classificatory system makes it more recognizable that all human beings are impaired in some way, will become acutely impaired at some time during the life course, and can become disabled in different ways by different environments.

There has also been much work in health and medical sociology which examines how the concept of health and related social phenomenon are profoundly changing; they are becoming 'diffused' beyond a scientific or disease focus, beyond the individual body and outside of the medical care system (Turner, 2004; Cribb, 2005; Blaxter, 2010). All of this is to say that the concept of health is profoundly changing; it is not exclusively focused on the absence of disease and is moving towards a holistic view. However, rather than sidestep the debates or muddle along with a nebulous concept of health, I am advancing a concept of health in relation to two fixed points in the literature and debates on the definition of health. I have triangulated my argument with Christopher Boorse's and Nordenfelt's theories of health as the former represents the prevailing though flawed view and the latter is what I consider to be the most coherent alternative. I am not alone in thinking that Boorse's and Nordenfelt's theories of health are the most important in the philosophy of health and medicine debates (Schramme, 2007). Though Boorse himself seems to think that there are four worthy challengers (Boorse, 2004). And lastly, I am not the first one to believe that capabilities theory can productively inform the conceptualization of health. Ian Law and Heather Widdows recently described the affinity between different accounts of health and the capabilities approach though they conclude that it requires further exploration and elaboration (Law and Widdows, 2008).

Conclusion

This chapter has reviewed Boorse's bio-statistical theory of health, Nordenfelt's theory of health and, lastly, has advanced a theory of health as being able to achieve ten central human functionings. Bringing together Nordenfelt's analysis with that of the CA has benefits for both. For Nordenfelt, his definition can become defensible by incorporating an idea of basic human capabilities and justifiable through freestanding ethical reasoning. For the CA, Nordenfelt provides a link to the philosophy of health debates and offers a way of avoiding getting waylaid by using the notion of health as the absence of disease. This is precisely the problem that Nussbaum faces with how she defines the health capability on her list. Also, the problems of ranking the basic capabilities and the unclear separation between the capability of living a long lifespan from the capability to be healthy get solved. Through health as a meta-capability, all the capabilities are recognized as being part of a cluster and inter-dependent.

Furthermore, some have argued that a non-scientific or ethical definition of health usually collapses into a conception of total well-being (Brock, 2002). Nordenfelt presents an argument for how health can be defined as a minimal account of well-being, or achieving vital goals. Rather than separate out a core set of physiological functionings as being health functionings from a complete set of well-being functionings, Nordenfelt's argument combined with Nussbaum's reasoning helps to define health as minimal conception of human well-being. Nordenfelt provides the structure of health as the ability to achieve vital goals for minimal happiness that includes both subjective and objective content of vital goals, while Nussbaum provides the content of the vital goals in the form of ten central human capabilities. The breadth and extent of these capabilities reflect a conception of human dignity that encompasses the neediness, sociability and ability to reason in pursuing a life plan.

As I said in the Introduction, a person's health and longevity is determined by the independent and interactive influences of her changing biological endowments and needs, external social and physical conditions, and her behaviours or agency. These components are the causal factors of health capability as well as human capabilities in general. Remember that health capability is a cluster of basic capabilities, and is a sub-set of all human capabilities. The focus in this chapter has been on conceptualizing health as the abilities to achieve a set of capabilities and functionings. The focus in the next chapter will be on the causal components of such capabilities. The main points to take away from this chapter are that the health as a concept can be defensibly conceived as a meta-capability, the capability to achieve a cluster of basic capabilities to be and do things that reflect a life worthy of equal human dignity. And, in case it needs emphasizing, Nordenfelt provides an independent line of reasoning to conceptualizing health as the ability to achieve a set of vital goals, which, I have argued, is the same as saying having the capability to achieve a set of basic functionings.

While Nussbaum grounds her 'vital capabilities' in human dignity, equal respect and other ethical values, Nordenfelt arrives at his vital goals or minimally decent life through linguistic and action-theory philosophy. And as I stated earlier, Nordenfelt is not the only individual seeking to define health in terms of abilities to function in the world. There are many other ways to get to health as an assessment of individual capabilities. All these ways of getting to a capability to be healthy thus bolster an argument operating from within the CA for a capability to be healthy.

Lastly, Nordenfelt's notion of health as the achieving of vital goals really brings to the forefront the notion of the primacy of health in the lives of individuals and societies. If achieving vital goals is indeed the most important thing in people's lives, then they should be the most important social goals. When Nordenfelt's reasoning is combined with Nussbaum's argument that the ten basic capabilities of citizens form the core of basic political principles, the reasoning further catapults health of citizens to the forefront of the social agenda. Philosophers and government officials often point out that health is only one among many pressing social goals, and individuals value health as only one among many other things in their life. They point to trade-offs that individuals are willing to make between health and other goods such as income. This view largely evidences the notion of health as the absence of disease. The priority of avoiding disease or impairments is not the same thing as the priority of health. When health is properly understood as achieving vital goals, and the entitlements to the capabilities of achieving these vital goals are duly recognized as basic political principles grounded in freedom and equal dignity, the health of citizens does become the first priority of social justice, and one of the most basic values of society.

2

Causation and Distribution of Health

I stated in the Introduction that a theory of health justice should have a coherent conception of health and the capacity to explain how it is created and distributed among individuals and groups. It would not be particularly helpful if an argument for health-related claims, even if not aspiring to be a full theory, did not have a coherent conception of health or relied on a muddled theory of causation and distribution of health. It is often with the implicit understanding that individual health cannot be created or distributed like money and other commodities that claims or a right to health are often summarily dismissed. Instead, discussion moves to possible claims to healthcare. So, if indeed, we are trying to make a case for claims to health, or health capability, then there is a burden to show how health is created and distributed. But aside from conceptual coherence in ethical discussions, for the social realization of health justice to be realistically possible, these arguments also have to be seen as being reasonable by individuals who work in health professions or by those who have the power to make health policy; there must be sufficient inter-theoretic coherence across the domain of ethics and the health disciplines. Moreover, as part of the method of justifying our considered moral judgements about health claims we have to confront and reconcile arguments about health claims with relevant sociological, epidemiological and biological facts and theories. That is what this chapter aims to do.

In Chapter 1, taking Boorse's theory as the best example of its kind, I criticised and rejected the supposedly factual or objective account of health as the most frequently occurring functionings in an age–sex reference class, and not limited by an environmental agent. I offered an alternative ethical conception of health as a meta-capability, a capability to achieve a cluster of vital goals or basic capabilities to be and do certain things. I also argued that Nussbaum's ten CHCs are a good start for such a cluster of basic capabilities and functionings which is applicable across the human species, thus creating a human species-wide conception of health. In the Introduction, I also sketched out that a human being's health and her capability to be healthy is made up of the interaction of an individual's biological endowments and needs, external social and physical environments and her behaviours.

As a result, I have so far in this book provided a rough account of a human capability, and a conception of health as a meta-capability to achieve a cluster of basic capabilities and functionings. In this chapter, my aim is provide a theory or account of the causation and distribution of capabilities and functionings, and relate this to our current, prevailing theories explaining the causation and distribution of health. The motivation for this is to argue that a theory of the causation and distribution of health capabilities should be the dominant paradigm in epidemiology. It overcomes many of the limitations of the current bio-medical paradigm, has many of the qualities that have been called for in a 'new epidemiology', and can bring together again the analysis of the health of all human beings within one framework. The last point is particularly important if we truly aim to build a meaningful framework for understanding and managing global health.

Rejecting the bio-medical model

As I said earlier, epidemiology is the informational engine of medical care and public health. And the prevailing disciplinary paradigm in epidemiology is substantively linked to the notion of disease. That is, most epidemiologists study the causation, frequency and distribution of disease. Consequently, rejecting the bio-statistical theory of health, which is centred on disease and prevalent in the health sciences, has implications for its counterpart 'biomedical' and multiple 'risk factor' theory of causation and distribution of disease currently dominant in the discipline of epidemiology. In the first instance, if we are expanding the concept of health beyond disease to the ability to achieve and exercise some basic capabilities, then we also want epidemiology to expand in order to study the causation and the distribution of basic capabilities. However, the capacity for the dominant paradigm in epidemiology simply to expand from examining disease determinants to capability determinants seems unfeasible. This chapter discusses why this is so and offers an alternative paradigm.

Along with the BST of health, the dominant biomedical and risk factor model of disease causation and distribution must also be rejected, or at least demoted, because it is inadequate as a general theory governing epidemiology. Lest I mislead, the demotion of the biomedical model in epidemiology is not primarily because it focuses too narrowly on the causation and distribution of disease. Rather, it is because as it currently stands, the dominant explanatory model in epidemiology is significantly constrained even in explaining diseases. It is not able to explain fully the causation and distribution of diseases most prevalent in developed economies, namely chronic and degenerative conditions. The current paradigm is not providing satisfactory explanations for all the observable facts of disease and its social distribution patterns.

Leonard Syme, one of epidemiology's most eminent teachers and researchers describes this situation as a crisis. As evidence for the need for a new paradigm, he points to the fact that after decades and millions of dollars put into research seeking to identify the risk factors for heart disease, even after putting together all the commonly accepted as well as the less accepted findings on risk factors, the totality of factors would still only explain about 40 per cent of cases (Syme, 1996). While some believe that the remaining 60 per cent of cases are likely to be explained by still-to-be-discovered genetic risk factors, Syme and others argue that it is the larger explanatory framework that is inadequate. Even if genes do have influence, rather than being completely deterministic, the surrounding environment influences how the genes express themselves. Our continued inability to identify comprehensively the causes of many chronic diseases is seen to be the fault of the explanatory paradigm used in epidemiology; not that we have yet to discover the cause through existing frameworks and methods of research.

Three specific limitations of the prevailing model of disease aetiology are often at the centre of debates about the 'paradigm crisis' in epidemiology. These include its level of analysis, its inability to recognize distribution patterns, and its partially informed recommendations for policy. The current model, which evolved from the late nineteenth-century germ theory of disease, recognizes three categories of causal factors. These factors include biological endowments, behaviours and external exposures to harmful substances or 'agents'. The resulting limitation of this model is that it operates only on a single level, at the individual level, and expresses a form of explanatory individualism. Short causal pathways confined to the human body are studied, while the model precludes recognizing any supra-individual level factors or social processes as part of the longer causal chain in the production of disease. As a result, the model studies individuals in a vacuum and disconnected from other individuals; it is focused only on what happens on and within the skin of individuals.

Furthermore, populations are understood as just a collection of individuals with no emergent properties. Therefore, public or population health is just the summation of the health of individuals. An individual, proximate factor analysis is restricted in recognizing the longer causal pathways to disease in individuals and restricted in recognizing the causal factors of disease distribution in populations (Rose, 1985; Wilkinson, 1996; Kelly et al., 2010).

The second limitation of the model is that it can only recognize certain patterns of distribution of disease and mortality across human beings. Because it can only group individuals according to biological features, behaviours, or external exposures, it has no internal source of information for grouping individuals by any other characteristics namely, social characteristics. Grouping individuals according to social characteristics in this model would be seen as unscientific and political (Murray et al., 1999a; Braveman et al., 2001). Thus, the inability to group individuals according to social features precludes the model's ability to analyse the possible causal impact of social conditions. This is because we would need first to identify differences among social groups in order to find social causes of the differences, just as we look for differences between people who have a disease and those who do not have disease in order to identify the cause. If only one particular social group cutting across age and sex got a particular disease, then it would be more plausible to separate by social groups. That would be based on the implicit understanding that some factor about this social group compared to other social groups related to biology, behaviour or exposures is causing disease in members of the social group. But, when we are concerned by inequalities – that a certain social group is affected more by a given disease than another – comparing social groups is seen to be an illegitimate analysis within epidemiology. Epidemiology is interested in what causes diseases in human beings as organisms, not why disease is distributed unevenly in historically contingent and culturally specific social groups. The concern over distribution appears to be 'normative', as it is about inequality, while the search for causation in individuals is seen to be scientific.

This view, however, misses out the possibility that a cause both creates a 'proximate' cause of disease in individuals and provides different amounts of exposure to different social groups. Moreover, the inability to analyse health outcomes by social groups within an epidemiological model means that the concern for health inequalities across social groups is pushed out of the disciplinary borders; it is seen as a sociological question rather than an epidemiological one.

The third limitation of the current model is that an explanatory model with restricted explanatory power and with limited capacity to recognize distribution patterns will prescribe only partially informed – and consequently incompletely effective – health policies.

While these are three very clear informational limitations that motivate searching for a better explanatory model, there are further ethical problems in continuing to adhere to an inadequate explanatory paradigm in epidemiology. If the explanatory model cannot explain the causation and distribution of certain diseases and cases of mortality, then we will come to view these cases as being beyond social action. We will come to see them as tragic cases that may compel acting with compassion, charity or pity. However, if the explanatory model is faulty, or we know it is inadequate and yet we continue to rely on it to guide our social responses, then we are likely to be committing moral errors by misidentifying cases as being tragic, even though they may be socially preventable or amenable. Injustice occurs twice in this situation.

Possible health injustice lies not only in the initial social causation of preventable impairments and mortality but again in neglecting to act, recognize, prevent or alleviate impairments and mortality. Carrying on using an explanatory model that we know is not fully robust and misclassifies causes as beyond social action would be showing supreme indifference and disrespect to those individuals whose impairments and mortality could be prevented if we had a better explanatory model. The pursuit of a better explanatory model is not only a matter of intellectual virtues of scientists; in the case of epidemiologists it is also an ethical obligation.

Epidemiology as a discipline has a unique role in social justice; it is not a science that is pursued purely for the sake of knowledge. It is an instrumental science that flows from the value we give to human health and longevity. Epidemiology provides the facts about the causes, levels, consequences, distributions and possible responses to impairments and mortality, which then are morally evaluated in order to determine social action. Continuing to adhere to an explanatory paradigm that is known to be inadequate and to misclassify or obscure certain types of causes not only diminishes the intellectual integrity of conducting science but also violates the dignity and moral claims of those individuals who suffer avoidable impairments and death. Because of the crucial importance knowledge of the causation and distribution of health and longevity has in the evaluation and realization of social justice, the institutions of epidemiology should be recognized as part of the basic structure of modern society alongside other basic social institutions such as legal courts and markets.

Norman Daniels has put forward such an argument in regard to medical care and public health programmes (Daniels, 1985). But these institutions are shaped and driven by epidemiology, and the moral importance we give to healthcare institutions in pursuing social justice is fundamentally reliant on epidemiology. Remember that hospitals and medical care only gained their reputation as being helpful after the underlying research became productive. Epidemiology provides the what, where, when, and how to provide medical care and public health programmes. Rather than simply thinking of the paradigm crisis in epidemiology as a problem of scientific theories concerning scientists – because the object of study is human health and longevity – we should see the paradigm crisis as a problem for a basic institution of social justice being faced by individuals who are primary agents of social justice. Imagine a court system that only functioned correctly 40 per cent of the time. We would not consider that as being a problem only for the lawyers and judges but as a problem for the whole of society. Similarly, epidemiology only producing sufficient explanations 40 per cent of the time is a problem for the whole society, since the freedom and dignity of individuals is at stake.

The current biomedical model is also likely to be constrained in explaining health because it is not able to explain sufficiently the causation and distribution of chronic and degenerative diseases. That is even if disconnected from the absence of disease notion, and focused instead on health as the most frequently occurring functionings in an age–sex reference class not limited by environmental agents, it would still have trouble. The limitations regarding levels of analysis, distribution patterns and partially informed solutions still would remain. Therefore, the possibility of the biomedical model being able to integrate or underwrite the idea of a capability to be healthy, conceived as opportunity or capabilities of achieving some basic functionings, seems even more far removed. So, for both informational and ethical reasons as well as the need to search for a counterpart epidemiological theory to the the conception of health as a meta-capability, the current biomedical model of disease causation has to be demoted because of its inherent limitations. I say demoted because the model is not always wrong. Sometimes, impairment is caused by individual-level, proximate factors such as physical exposures, behaviours or genetic traits. Yet, because of its informational limitations and propagation of moral errors such as misclassifying disease and mortality as being outside of social action and obscuring social inequalities in health, it must be replaced by a better explanatory paradigm. We need a general theory in epidemiology that is not only more robust in explaining the causation and distribution of all diseases but also in explaining the causation and distribution of health, properly conceived.

New epidemiology and capabilities theory

Others with significantly more expertise in epidemiology than I have previously argued that a new kind of epidemiology has to emerge that can bring together micro-analyses such as molecular biology with social science that examines the most macro-perspectives (Susser, 1999). The notion is that we need to integrate analyses from micro to macro and the natural with the social sciences in order to identify the causation and distribution of disease and premature mortality. We need to link individual level phenomena with population level phenomena (Kelly et al., 2010). I believe that there is much affinity between what Mervyn Susser outlines as 'multidimensional epidemiology' that is now required and a theory of the causation and distribution of human capabilities. In proposing a new multi-dimensional theory for epidemiology, I bring together the most recent work in social epidemiology that explodes outward the current biomedical model in order to study social determinants of disease together with the 'entitlement analysis' of famines undertaken by Jean Drèze and Amartya Sen.

This may initially strike some as peculiar, but there is much to learn from bringing together social epidemiology and the study of acute and endemic malnutrition. The entitlement analysis, which is a social science analysis of malnutrition, is the precursor to modern capabilities theory. And, unlike heuristic or mathematical models of capabilities, the entitlement analysis focuses on embodied human beings and their capability to achieve adequate nutrition. I believe it illuminates how to bring biology and social science together to explain health capabilities as well as how deftly to demote a longstanding and dominant yet inadequate explanatory paradigm.

Staying true to the claim that that this book presents an inter-disciplinary argument, what follows is a review of the evolution and content of modern social epidemiology; it is a bit of history and philosophy of science. I focus largely on social epidemiology rather than on recent advances in epidemiological study design, data analysis or particular areas such as molecular epidemiology for two reasons. I want to reinforce the reasons why the individual level model is insufficient and does not present the complete causal picture by presenting evidence of supra-individual level causal factors. Second, this book is centrally aimed at creating wider appreciation of the profound social bases of the causation and distribution of disease and mortality as well as pointing to the breadth of possibilities of social action that could be directed at the causes, persistence, levels and consequences of ill-health and mortality.

There are many recent developments in epidemiology that are noteworthy, but they do not overcome the three limitations of the individual level, biomedical model. In contrast, social epidemiology is attempting to break the constraints of the biomedical model and connects molecular biology with social science. And, by showing the underlying affinity between social epidemiology and the entitlement analysis/capabilities approach I aim to explode out social epidemiology even further to the most macro-perspective. And conversely, I aim to ground capabilities theory in the physical and mental functionings of embodied human beings.

After reviewing some of the seminal findings and research topics in social epidemiology, I argue for a 'unified theory' of health causation and distribution that can bring together analyses from the molecular level to global political economy, integrating natural and social sciences, as well as one that can integrate how we understand and respond to the health issues faced by individuals in rich and poor countries. As a companion theory to a conception of health as a capability that is applicable to every member of the human species, the theory of causation and distribution of health capabilities can also be seen to be coherent for all human beings. Coming up with a new paradigm for epidemiology is undoubtedly an incredibly ambitious goal. And, I would not attempt to suggest such a project were it not for the fact that I am standing on the shoulders of giants.

The main advocates of the capabilities approach have already done much over the past three decades to argue that capabilities theory should be a general theory of human well-being across all societies, rich and poor, East and West. What I am arguing is that a small part of that general theory of capabilities, which deals with 'basic capabilities', should be the dominant paradigm in epidemiology. Significant work in other social science disciplines, particularly econometrics, is already underway to develop models that assist in measuring the causes, distribution and dynamics of capabilities (Chiappero-Martinetti and Roche, 2009). There is already some work underway in measuring Nussbaum's ten capabilities within the health context (Coast et al., 2008a).

What I am doing is making a modest link between the search for a better explanatory paradigm in epidemiology with an extant global theory of human well-being framed in terms of capabilities. A theory of the causation and distribution of basic human capabilities could plausibly be a multi-dimensional theory of epidemiology that can account for causal factors from the molecular to the global, assess health issues facing individuals in all countries whether rich or poor, and provide comprehensive information about distribution patterns. Moreover, the ethical arguments regarding justice and capabilities provide guidance on social action. That is the focus of Parts II and III of the book. More presently is the discussion of the empirical theories of causation and distribution of disease and health.

Theories of disease causation and distribution

William H. Stewart, the highest ranking medical official in United States government in the 1960s, is often quoted as having said during his tenure as US Surgeon General that it was 'time to close the book on infectious diseases' (Mann et al., 1992, p. 825; Bristol, 2008). Whether or not this is an accurate attribution, the quote nicely reflects the triumphalism among medical and public health professionals at that time. Late nineteenth-century and post-war scientific advances including microscopy, germ theory, bacteriology and the development of vaccines and antibiotics were credited with dramatically curtailing premature deaths and impairments due to infectious diseases in industrialized countries.

Moreover, by the early 1970s it was believed that all infectious diseases and effective methods to contain them had been identified. The continuing spread of infectious diseases in poor or non-industrialized countries was attributed to abject poverty, over-population and poor governance; conditions not dissimilar to those in pre-industrialized Europe and America. Indeed, based on the experience of the

United Kingdom and the United States, theories of demographic and epidemiologic transitions were proposed to explain how societies achieve better health through economic development or how during the process of industrialization societies move from experiencing infectious diseases and high fertility and mortality to chronic diseases and stable populations (Omran, 1971; Preston, 1975). By the late 1960s and early 1970s, the achievements of modern medical science and healthcare were undoubtedly compelling. With the control of infectious diseases, the focus in the second half of the twentieth century was to be on non-infectious diseases such as heart disease, cancers and strokes, as these were now the largest cause of premature mortality and impairments in the United States and other developed economies.

In moving away from studying infectious diseases towards chronic diseases a variety of methods were developed to identify the aetiology of disease; these included case-control methods, cohort studies and, starting in the 1970s, researchers began using computers to carry out increasingly complex statistical calculations on large data sets (Saracci, 2010). In contrast to the single causative agent central to germ theory, the basic paradigm since the first textbooks on epidemiological methods were published in the mid twentieth century is that of 'multiple causation'. The multi-factoral causation model hypothesizes a chain of different factors encompassing exposures to hazardous materials, genetic endowments or 'predispositions', and behaviours (MacMahon et al., 1960; Krieger, 1994; Rothman et al., 2008).

Importantly, the first epidemiology textbook published in the United States proposed understanding the multiple factor aetiology of disease in the following way (MacMahon et al., 1960; Susser, 1985). The authors argued that a linear, causal chain of multiple factors does not take into account the complex precursors to each component of the chain, and that the precursors and chain components might overlap or have interactions creating a variety of direct and indirect effects on the progression to disease. The authors advised eschewing the old notion of a single agent or a serial chain of events causing disease and proposed an understanding of causality of disease metaphorically envisioned as the 'web of causation'. The web model, according to the authors, also benefited from not having to prioritize different causal factors, and focused attention instead on identifying the determinants that are both necessary for disease and most amenable to intervention. The epidemiologist's objective is to identify the most *proximate* link in the web to the disease in order to cut the links (MacMahon et al., 1960; Krieger, 1994).

Both Susser and Nancy Krieger write that this web of causation has been a very influential metaphor governing the epistemology of modern epidemiology. Krieger, in particular, aims to highlight how the metaphor and the consequent methodology exclude many causal factors or links in the web. In an influential essay entitled, 'Where is the spider?' she tracks how the analysis of social factors was excluded in the evolution of the web of causation theory and focused narrowly on individual and proximate factors (Krieger, 1994). The web of causation model of MacMahon and colleagues presents a theoretical framework that subscribes to health individualism, and emphasizes acting on proximate determinants of disease amenable to intervention through individual level healthcare or technological interventions and individual behaviour change. It considers supra-individual factors or social determinants to be second-order, distal factors that are possibly irrelevant to preventing disease in individuals. And lastly, it sees the population distribution of diseases as simply a sum of individual cases of disease. Krieger observes that, 'In this view, disease in populations is reduced to a question of disease in individuals, which in turn is reduced to a question of biological malfunctioning' (Krieger, 1994, p. 892). The biomedical view of population health is simply the aggregate picture of biological malfunctioning of individuals.

This model of biological or health individualism that has come to dominate epidemiology has been fundamentally shaped by the social context in the United States during the second half of the twentieth century. In particular, Krieger argues that the exclusion of social factors from the scope of epidemiology and academic discourses on disease causation resulted from the political environment of the Cold War which curtailed examination of social class and social inequalities (Krieger, 1994, p. 890). Anti-communist fervour restricted open research as well as engendered self-censorship in examining the impact of social conditions in disease causation. Also, the push to make social sciences more like the natural sciences, seen to be objective and value free, exerted pressure on epidemiologists to focus on biomedical and individual focused factors.

Meanwhile, in the United Kingdom, where epidemiology first developed as method of enquiry, the concern over social class inequalities in mortality and impairments was a prominent public concern post Second World War. There was a visible public worry over social inequality and poverty, particularly the deprivation of the worst-off in society (Szreter, 1984). Starting in 1913, the government of the United Kingdom officially recognized and began analysing health progress by the social category of socio-economic class (Szreter, 1984). Social position or class was defined by five groupings of occupations which were said to reflect not only income, but also similar culture and social status. This classification was not without problems but, unlike using data stratified by sex, age or residence, this classification system allowed the recognition of differences in mortality and its rate of progress across socio-economic classes over time.

The common opinion in Britain during the 1950s and 1960s was that the dramatic improvement in life expectancy and morbidity that was markedly visible at the beginning of the century would continue unabated. The creation of the National Health Service (NHS), which provided free healthcare to all, was meant to ensure that all parts of society would share in the health improvements. The NHS was meant to alleviate inequalities both in access to healthcare – that was a clear problem under the previous private medical care system – as well as inequalities in health achievements across the socio-economic classes. The persistence of higher mortality rates and slower progress among the poorest classes during the 1950s and 1960s was made visible because of the use of class in the census data was attributed to a time lag. That is to say, the better-off and educated were understood to be more likely to be the first to take advantage of new information or technology, thus there would be a time lag before everybody takes advantage of the resources and benefit.

The Black Report and Whitehall studies

As in most other industrialized countries, the leading causes of mortality and impairments in post Second World War Britain were degenerative diseases related to ageing and non-communicable chronic diseases such as heart disease, cancers and strokes. By the 1960s, the transition from high mortality rates due to infectious diseases to lower mortality rates due to chronic conditions had become well established,resulting in the entire British population living longer than previous generations. However, the persistence of higher rates of premature mortality among the lowest socio-economic classes well into the 1970s could no longer be explained away as simply being due to a time lag. After taking account of war-related mortality, even after decades of functioning government welfare programmes and provision of free healthcare, there were still higher premature mortality rates and disease precursors in the lower social classes. This concern for the health of the lowest socio-economic classes moved the British government to establish a Working Group on Health Inequalities (WGHI) in 1977 (Black et al., 1992). The remit of the working group was to review the aggregate differences in health achievements between socio-economic classes, evaluate the possible causes, identify implications for government policy, and identify areas and questions requiring further research.

The final report of that committee released in 1980, known as the Black Report, has proven to be a watershed event for initiating public debate not only in Britain but world wide about social inequalities in health. It also motivated a whole new area of health research on the causation of inequalities in impairments and longevity across social groups (Black et al., 1992; Macintyre, 1997; Whitehead, 1998).

Though the Black Report uses the term 'health' the WGHI chose to focus only on mortality rates in order to avoid the difficulties with the complexity of the concept of health. The WGHI simply took biological viability or ability to stay alive as the irreducible absolutist core of the idea of health. Thus, in actuality, the working group examined the unequal distribution of longevity across British citizens stratified by age, sex and socio-economic class. Inequalities in health meant inequalities in length of lifespans. And to this day, the rhetoric of inequalities in health or the social determinants of health actually refers to the social determinants and inequalities in disease and premature mortality.

The WGHI reviewed four possible explanations for the persistence of higher mortality among the lower classes. The explanatory categories encompassed the full range of extant aetiological theories ranging from the biological, behavioural and environmental. What is worth noting is that the categories of explanations the WGHI considered shows that the core debates on the aetiology and distribution of ill-health in the late twentieth century were remarkably similar to those in the late nineteenth century.

Making use of nascent forms of empirical analysis, nineteenth-century British and French researchers had postulated that the higher rates of premature mortality and impairments among the lower social classes were due to inherent biological characteristics of individuals (genetic quality), their volitional behaviours (culture of poverty), or factors in the environment shaped by social and economic structures (material poverty). Aetiological theories which concentrated on individual level biological pathways such as miasma or germ theories competed with these other explanations. The spectacular success of germ theory in reducing mortality at the turn of the twentieth century fully undermined miasma theory, and also muted advocacy for the three other alternative theories.

However, the persistence of premature morality and social inequalities in health in the later twentieth century rejuvenated the theories posited in the previous century, though they reappeared in slightly different guises. Interestingly, the issue at stake in the modern debates seemed to be almost identical to the one prominent prior to the rise of germ theory namely, why do the lower socio-economic classes or 'the poor' die younger and experience more disease?

The four categories of causal explanations for the socio-economic class differences or inequalities in mortality that were examined included:

Artefact explanations. These explanations asserted that there was no relation between social class and health, but that they were simply measurement errors due to the changing population structures.

Theories of natural or social selection. In this conception, the inability of the poor to stay alive or free from disease indicated their weaker status as human organisms, and thus determined their lower social class position. A less stringent hereditary/eugenics position was that people who are ill or disabled move down in occupations associated with the lower classes.

Materialist or structural explanations. These theories posited that economic and associated socio-structural factors determined physical susceptibility as well as exposure to hazards in the housing and work environment. Poverty in the form of material deprivation directly resulted in premature mortality and morbidity.

Cultural/behavioural explanations. This category asserted that the unthinking, reckless and irresponsible behaviour of individuals such as excessive drinking and sexual promiscuity were predominant in the lower classes, and associated with high mortality and morbidity.

After three years of deliberation, the WHGI concluded that persistence of higher mortality among the poorer classes was largely due to 'materialist and structural' causes. The recommendations emphasized increasing the role of health services sector, and implementing a broad anti-poverty strategy. Sally Macintyre writes that the debates after the release of the Black Report suggest that though the material and structural explanation was identified as the main cause it was without sufficient justification or explication of the causal pathways (Macintyre, 1997). Her analysis is that materialist explanation was selected mainly because it was the only category left after dismissing the three other alternative explanations.

Moreover, Macintyre then goes on to say that the Report's recommendations for improving education, addressing health damaging behaviours, and helping disabled individuals reflected the committee affirming a 'soft' version of each of the other explanations as well (Macintyre, 1997). So the Black Report rejected the social class differences in mortality as being due to artefact, but accepted some role of all the other factors which can roughly be reduced to biology, behaviour, and external social and material environment.

However nuanced the recommendations of the WGHI may have been, the general conclusion that significant public resources would need to be spent to improve the health of the poorest classes was not well received by the newly elected Conservative government. The government attempted to suppress the Black Report in a variety of ways (Black et al., 1992). Nevertheless, partly due to the academic credentials of the committee members, the Black Report's conclusions were publicized by the media, health academic community, and the shadow government. As a result, the report has had a profound impact on the scope and nature of public debate on health, health research and poverty alleviation which continues to the present day in the United Kingdom and beyond.[1]

The Black Report's concern over social inequalities in health achievements, particularly longevity, was significantly bolstered by the findings from a 1978 study looking at the health of 17,530 British civil servants known as the Whitehall Study (Marmot et al., 1978). What started out as a conventional study of the risk factors for cardiovascular and respiratory disease among a large, defined and accessible population of research subjects produced startling findings. The conventional thought at that time was that senior managers at the top of organizations were the most under stress and suffered more heart disease and mortality. Michael Marmot and colleagues reported results which showed the opposite. The individuals at the bottom of the organization had higher rates of mortality and disease. But what is most astounding is that the researchers found a clearly visible step-wise gradient in disease and mortality paralleling the rank of employment. Starting from the top grade, each rank of civil servants had worse health than the rank above. In comparison, the WGHI did not really focus on the gradient in mortality across the five socio-economic classes; it was focused largely on the higher mortality of the lower classes. Consequently, they advocated for social interventions that would address material deprivation of the worst-off or lowest social class.

The Whitehall study showed that even when absolute material deprivation is not a factor, as all civil service employees across all grade levels were above the threshold of poverty, there still was a social gradient in health right across all the employment grades. So, something else aside from material deprivation was influencing health. Initially the Whitehall researchers thought this pattern was only associated with the risk factors and prevalence of heart and respiratory disease. But the distribution pattern was confirmed across all diseases including gastrointestinal disease, renal disease, strokes, accidental mortality, violent mortality and cancers that were and were not related to smoking (Kreisler, 2002). Subsequent follow-up studies, ten and twenty-five years later, which also included women, showed that the step-wise pattern remained (Marmot et al., 1997, 1998).

This identification of a step-wise gradient in health indicators according to social position in a hierarchy, reflected by the civil service grade of employment, has also instigated a tremendous amount of research across the world on health inequalities. Perhaps as remarkable as the original study is that the social gradient in health was confirmed not only across the entire British population, but also across the populations in every industrialized society (Adler et al., 1994; Macintyre, 1997).

More recently, Marmot and colleagues have shown that such a gradient is also present in developing countries (World Health Organization and Commission on Social Determinants of Health, 2008). The Whitehall studies have resulted in a range of key findings about determinants of health and social inequalities in health. Aside from the uncontested causal role of material deprivation, biological risk factors, and individual behaviours, the studies clearly established that relative social position is correlated with health outcomes. Subsequent studies which controlled for individual behaviours, such as smoking and diet, showed individual behaviours could not explain the distribution; the social gradient still persists (Marmot et al., 2008). And other studies have shown that biological endowments or health conditions do not significantly influence which grade one ends up in the civil service. The Whitehall studies also show that contrary to common understanding, health achievements are not distributed dichotomously according to a threshold between the 'haves' and the 'have-nots'. Longevity and disease were distributed in a continuous social gradient.

Furthermore, by establishing a link between social conditions and ill-health and mortality and the social gradient in health outcomes, the studies highlighted the limitations of the classic biomedical model in epidemiology. The classic biomedical model's causal factors of biological endowment, individual behaviours, and exposures to harmful agents could not fully explain the ill-health of individuals, and the step-wise gradient (Marmot, 2004a, 2004b; Siegrist and Marmot, 2004; Marmot, 2006).

The Whitehall research has generated the hypothesis that a social cause can distribute the harmful exposure to different social groups differently, while also being the cause of disease in individuals. So, for example, social arrangements determining the nature of the food supply, food culture, food prices, and availability also determine which social groups are exposed to which foods. Individuals in certain social groups become directly exposed to foods high in saturated fats and salt, which leads to high cholesterol and blood pressure, causing heart disease. The variety of social arrangements that determine the dietary intake of fatty and salty foods by an individual are referred to as 'the causes of the cause'. The causes of the causes distribute the level of exposures to different social groups. This way of looking at causation has significant implications for standard epidemiology, which often focuses on biological markers as causes of disease; in this case blood plasma cholesterol and blood pressure would be seen as the risk factor or cause.

Rather than only focusing on the biology and behaviour of the individual, the 'cause of the cause' framework explodes out the causal model and causal chain. It follows the chain back temporally and upwards to supra-individual level factors. As a result, epidemiology and the study of health begin to look more like social science than natural science.

The Whitehall research has also expanded research into psycho-social processes such as those affected by workplace environment. Some of the Whitehall II studies suggest that the social gradient in mortality reflects an individual-level, psychosocial mechanism mediating between external social conditions and the production of disease within an individual (Marmot and Brunner, 1999). The 'infection' travels through psychobiological pathways. An individual's 'control', 'agency', 'dignity', and how fairly individuals are treated, as well as how interesting they find their work, have been suggested as aspects of the workplace which differ according to employment grade and may be correlated to the gradient in health outcomes (Kreisler, 2002). The expectation is that such workplace features can be extrapolated to other environments such as the home and community (Syme and Balfour, 1997).

Causation theories and social epidemiology

In the pursuit of causal pathways between social determinants and mortality and disease across individuals and social groups, the classic, biomedical model of disease causation has been overlaid or stretched in various ways. The social environment is seen as the missing 'spider' in the web of causation and is included in the models as another variable. But what become immediately apparent is the ubiquity of the influence of the social on health and longevity. Social determinants influence genetic endowments by determining who is conceived and how their genetic traits are expressed; they influence social processes that work directly through psychobiological pathways; they influence or shape individual behaviours; they determine the physical or material environment. In essence, all three factors of the classic biomedical model have a social precursor, and so all epidemiology could be considered to be social epidemiology. While this indeed may be true, and there is a need for a general theory for epidemiology, specific areas of research have flourished over the past three decades making use of existing analytical resources. Research has been done on such determinants as psychosocial pathways, political-economy, income inequality, social capital and life course experience.

Psychosocial theories

In what is regarded an important milestone in social epidemiology, John Cassel presented a lecture to the American Public Health Association in 1976 on the need to address the psychosocial factors that decrease biological resistance to disease through better identification and categorization of factors at the social level rather than at the individual level (Cassel, 1976). Cassel stated that two important findings regarding the body's responses to stressors needed to be recognized. First, biological processes that regulate susceptibility to disease were weakened when an actor does not perceive evidence that her actions are resulting in the intended consequences. The second finding was that the biological responses to stress-inducing situations were ameliorated by the strength of the social support provided by other people considered as being important by the individual.

There was much debate and discussion following Cassel's lecture that considered a range of issues, including whether animal research from which these psychosocial effects were identified were applicable to human beings; if it is possible to carry out ethical experiments on humans to test these ideas; to what extent the biological mechanisms had been sufficiently specified; and whether stress creates a general susceptibility or if particular biological responses to stress lead to susceptibility to specific diseases.

At about the same time, Marmot with Leonard Syme, one of the pioneers and early teachers of social epidemiology, were examining the possible influence of social factors on health by comparing the health status of Japanese male immigrants to the United States and a counterpart group of men residing in Japan. The research showed that Japanese immigrants took on the disease profile of the surrounding White American population. This undermined the emphasis on the inherent biological basis of health profiles. If groups have inherent biological characteristics, Japanese men should have the same health profile anywhere they live. But the studies showed that was not the case, and even more. Those Japanese immigrants who were more assimilated into the surrounding American community experienced more of the diseases affecting the majority White population. These findings supported the thesis that health profiles are not purely determined by genetics or individual behaviours but also by surrounding social environments (Marmot and Syme, 1976). Cassel's lecture as well as the more recent work of Marmot and colleagues point to various psychosocial determinants such as agency, control, stress and social support. These pathways are continuing to be conceptualized and researched (Marmot et al., 1999; Singh-Manoux, 2003).

Income inequality and health

Separate research carried out in the 1980s also complemented studies on psychosocial pathways. In a seminal article published in 1992, Richard Wilkinson began to show evidence that higher income inequality in societies was correlated with lower population average health and higher social inequalities in health (Wilkinson, 1992). The Wilkinson thesis shows that in countries above a threshold of $25,000 GNP per capita, larger average-income differences between classes are associated with a steeper gradient in health and higher overall mortality in the entire population (Wilkinson, 1997; Kawachi et al., 1999; Wilkinson, 2000). Below the threshold, income inequality shows no correlation with the gradient in health outcomes. He maintains that below the threshold, absolute material deprivation has more significant influence on mortality and health outcomes than income inequality.

Across a number of industrialized countries, and within regions of countries, Wilkinson's analysis shows that the steepness of the health gradient is associated with level of income inequality. More recently the research has linked income inequality with a wide range of social problems aside from steeper health gradient and lower health outcomes (Wilkinson and Pickett, 2009). While many have received this research as referring to material determinants of health, Wilkinson argues that the effect of income inequality lies first in the psychosocial effects of being of lower social status, experiencing subordination, or being denied respect (Wilkinson, 1996). Static as well as increasing income inequality affects social standing and in turn, leads to biological processes in the individual, such as chronic anxiety, permanent increases in stress hormones such as cortisol, more atherosclerosis and poorer immunity. The total result of these processes that occur through psychobiological pathways is said to be analogous to rapid ageing (Kawachi et al., 1999, p. 493).

Political economy

Aside from methodological critiques, a number of alternative explanations have been posited for the role of income inequality in the causation and distribution of premature mortality and impairments. One possibility is that a larger force such as broader social ideologies and cultural behaviours determines structures that result both in income inequalities and health inequalities. David Coburn, for example, argues that it is not simply income–inequality in a vacuum but the dominant ideology of neo-liberalism that is causing both the income inequality and health inequalities (Coburn, 2004).

Vincent Navarro maintains that politics and political regimes are directly implicated in the increasing health inequalities. He shows this through identifying the changes in health inequalities according to the political regimes in power. Looking specifically at infant mortality rates from 1945 to 1980 in developed, capitalist countries, Navarro finds that governments representative of labour movements and social democratic parties committed to redistributive policies showed better infant mortality rates than the more libertarian governments such as the United States and United Kingdom, where income inequality is more tolerated (Navarro, 1993; Navarro and Shi, 2001).

Leonard Syme offers more theoretical alternatives to Coburn and Navarro's empirical explanations for the income inequality and health inequality association (Syme, 1998). He hypothesizes that the well-off may be simply doing much better than the worse-off given that it is much harder for those at the bottom of a steep social hierarchy to achieve as much, if at all, compared with those at the top. Simply put, improved opportunities for health achievements accrue to those who are already able to take advantage of them. They have more agency. A second possible explanation is that the richer can simply acquire many more material goods that help them achieve better health.

A third explanation, based on animal studies, suggests relative deprivation is rooted in evolutionary biology. It posits that individuals in whatever environment will see themselves as having less and achieving less that those with more of whatever is the valued asset, whether it is income or bananas. Hierarchy will always be present and, therefore, so too will the consequent social gradient in health outcomes. Syme's final hypothesis is that individuals don't mind being worse-off if everyone is considered to be in the same situation, but become very troubled when they believe that others are better-off through unfair social arrangements. Steep income inequalities cause biological responses that produce ill-health because they are perceived as being unfair social conditions. It is not envy but a sense of injustice that causes biological processes that lead to ill-health.

In contrast to Syme's concern with hierarchy, income inequalities and health inequalities, Angus Deaton argues that social status 'in and of itself' does not produce any health benefit (Deaton, 2011). Only when the privileges or greater resources of those with higher social status have something to buy or use that improves health and longevity does the social gradient in health appear historically in the seventeenth century. And, importantly, the link between status and technology also underlies contemporary dynamics of health inequalities within countries and between countries. The first to benefit from new technologies or information regarding health tend to be the better-off and educated, thus exacerbating health inequalities. With appropriate social policy, such technologies should diffuse to the rest of the population after some time. It is the differences in social commitment to the broader provision of health technologies that can explain poor health and health inequalities (Sen, 2011). But Deaton recognizes that the link between social status and availability of health technologies provides only a part of the explanations for the social inequalities in health. In his most recent writings, he focuses on childhood inequalities as a source of many health inequalities and argues that societies would do well to break 'the injustice of parental circumstances determining children's outcomes' (Deaton, 2011).

Social capital

Aside from directly impacting on the individual's biological processes through psychological pathways, Wilkinson also identifies a second effect of income inequality, the dissipating of social cohesion. Increasing inequalities in income change the nature of social relations by decreasing levels of trust, increasing hostility and violence, dissipating social networks and increasing domestic conflict. This consequent 'culture of inequality' is starkly compared to the income egalitarian and cohesive community identified by Robert Putnam in his influential research on civic society in different regions of Italy (Putnam et al., 1993; Putnam, 2000). Bringing together Putnam's sociological analysis on social capital and Wilkinson's income inequality thesis, a number of researchers have found levels of trust, levels of hostility, and rates of homicide and violent crime have a strong correlation with these factors and income inequality (Kawachi et al., 1999).

The overlap between Wilkinson's underlying concern with social cohesion within his thesis on income inequality and Putnam's work on 'social capital' has motivated some researchers to examine directly the association between social cohesion and health outcomes. And Putnam himself remarked on the better health and longevity of those communities with more social capital. Putnam refers to social capital as the connections between individuals in the form of social networks and the norms of reciprocity and trustworthiness that arise from them. From analysing the historical and social changes in regions of Italy over a twenty-year period, and subsequently in America, Putnam argues that 'generalized reciprocity' within a small social group, community or an entire society can generate great social and economic benefits (Putnam et al., 1993; Putnam, 2000). Within the conception of social capital, Putnam identifies two different types of relationships. 'Bonding capital' refers to relationships among social groups made of individuals of similar background, and thus trust and reciprocity occurs without hesitation. 'Bridging capital' is relationships among individuals who may not share any common background characteristics but come together to undertake cooperative activity.

In reviewing Putnam's theory, particularly in relation to health inequalities, Simon Szreter argues for a greater inclusion of the role of the state, and also identifies the importance of what he terms 'linking capital', or the relationships between significantly unequal individuals and civic organizations on the one hand, and government institutions, on the other hand (Szreter, 2002).

Social capital analysis as a model for community development has become popular across many disciplines and institutions. Despite the rapid dispersion of the idea, and the application of the concept to health inequalities in particular, Macinko and Starfield conclude that there does not seem to be a consensus on the nature of social capital, and its appropriate level of analysis, or the appropriate means to measure it (Macinko and Starfield, 2001).

Wilkinson's thesis offers a pathway between income inequality, social cohesion and the impact on psychobiological processes. But, when starting at the community level with empirical measurements of social cohesion, and without any further evidence of how social cohesion is increased or decreased, it has proven less useful in explaining the aetiology or distribution of disease and mortality.

Interestingly, what social capital and health research has established is the idea that a particular community has health characteristics that can be observed in the same way as the presence of a particular type of environmental pollutant. The research treats the social determinants such as trust and reciprocity as a property of the social group. Since the initial studies looking at the social processes affecting health, a group of researchers have focused more on the idea of a place having influence on health. Various studies have shown how cities and neighbourhoods have identifiable effects on the health of individuals. That is, research shows the influence of place after accounting for existing health conditions, and individual behaviours (Subramanian and Kawachi, 2004).

Life course approach

Wilkinson contends that the effect of low social status or acute subordination resulting from income inequality as well as the existence of egalitarian relationships, in the form of ideal friendships, can have a profound effect early on in the life course. The transference of low status of parents to the development experience of the child, and the ability of the child to establish friendships during the early years of life, is hypothesized as greatly modulating the psychosocial effects of income inequality later in life (Kawachi et al., 1999). In a similar vein, a growing body of evidence is being presented that the health constraints experienced by adults may be significantly pre-programmed in infancy as well as in-utero. David Barker and colleagues show that a biological imprint on the human body occurs in the foetal and infant period impacted by the mother's health, which is particularly vulnerable in contexts of material deprivation (Barker, 1990, 1991). Low birth-weight and retardation of the foetus is linked to higher risk of adult onset of respiratory disease, diabetes, heart disease, stroke, and certain cancers (Vagero and Illsley, 1995). Barker writes that the geographical and social inequalities in mortality rates and impairments across the United Kingdom could be explained through the experience of poverty by mothers.

Other researchers have subsequently studied non-biological, early life pathways that result in adult health constraints (Vagero and Illsley, 1995). For example, social disadvantage early in life results in a series of denied opportunities – such as schooling, employment and marriage – and other negative experiences that cumulatively combine to produce disease starting in middle age. Along the same lines, Davey-Smith has argued that income inequality does not produce significant and immediate health conditions but instead, a lifetime of experience of low social status leading to an accumulation of biological effects that eventually lead to premature mortality and visible impairments in adulthood (Krieger and Davey Smith, 2004).

Though Barker's studies on early biological programming have opened an area of research on the life course perspective on health, his work has also come under much criticism (Vagero and Illsley, 1995). Marmot's scepticism of Barker's research relies partly on 'natural experiments' such as the remarkable differences in mortality rates of the former Austro-Hungarian countries after the Second World War. If indeed, there is biological programming in-utero, there would be a cohort effect across the now independent countries. But there is not. Instead, there is a significant divergence in the health of the Austrian population, which is considered part of Western Europe, and the health of populations of Hungary and Czechoslovakia, which are considered to be part of Eastern Europe. It is perhaps unnecessary to say that the mortality rates in Austria are much lower than in the other two countries. Marmot contends that the differing social and economic factors post independence, rather than biological programming in-utero, causes the significant differences and similarities in the three countries. He remarks further that the same sort of divergence which happened between the Eastern and Western Europe divide is probably what is causing the differences across different regions within countries such as the United Kingdom. And not, as Barker contends, due to geographical differences in deprivations experienced by pregnant women (Marmot et al., 1998).

Eco-social epidemiology

While epidemiologists are familiar with the term 'ecological' as referring to group-level analysis, and the 'ecological fallacy' of attributing to an individual the characteristics of the surrounding group, the 'eco-social' theory of health and illness is conceptualized as describing processes simultaneously occurring at multiple levels, starting from

DNA and going on through protein to organ to individual to community and beyond. The conceptualization of one level of processes nested into another has led to using the metaphor of 'Chinese boxes' to describe a possible new paradigm of epidemiology. The metaphor, perhaps more accurately a Japanese bento box, is deployed to show the inter-related and nested nature of biological processes. The Chinese box, it is argued, also aims to be a significant shift from the current 'black box' methodology where multiple, individual level factors are analysed for strength of association without an explication of the exact relationship (Susser and Susser, 1996b). Correlation is often assumed to be causation without identifying the pathway.

Though the eco-social model has only recently begun to be explored in epidemiology, Richard Levins and Richard Lowentin have been asserting since the 1970s and 1980s the need to replace unidirectional cause and effect theories with more complex models of the dialectical relationships between humans, other organisms, and the environment (Levins and Lewontin, 1985). Their eco-social theory of health is said to be informed by a variety of sources – most notably biology, agriculture, epidemiology, philosophy and systems theory (Levins and Lopez, 1999). Levins argues that current methodology of epidemiology has focused too narrowly on specific problems such as a single disease. Though the focus on a single disease can help to identify therapy for that particular disease, it obscures or ignores the much wider and larger issues in the causation and distribution of illness and mortality. For example, Levins makes the point that identifying and implementing a solution to a single disease, such as vertical health programmes, can have negative consequences on other processes that affect human mortality and impairments.

Levins further criticizes the multiple risk-factor epidemiological model which attempts to give relative weights to various factors in the causation of disease as being a victim of Cartesian reductivism. Large problems are broken down to individual parts, without recognizing the additional properties at the system level. He argues that rather than the either/or distinctions such as genetics/individual volition, individual/environment, and mind/body, a theory of health should incorporate all the factors in a complex system of analysis made up with more than unidirectional pathways and include feedback loops, time lags and other interactive relationships. The importance of systems analysis, first developed by biologists in the early twentieth century seems now to be being taken up in epidemiology in the form of non-linear models, such as the 'Chinese box' theory of disease causation (Krieger, 1994; Susser and Susser, 1996a, 1996b, Krieger, 2001).

Development and health

If one quickly reviews the literature on social epidemiology, it becomes fairly obvious that most of the research about social determinants of health has been done in developed economies. The lack of social determinants research in developing countries appears to evidence Deaton's argument that the better-off often benefit from new technologies first. Indeed, the recent report of the WHO Commission on the Social Determinants of Health argued that social determinants of health and health inequalities affect all countries (World Health Organization and Commission on Social Determinants of Health, 2008). But such an effort to globalize the concern for social determinants of health appears to be weakened by research coming from within social epidemiology. For example, Wilkinson's thesis is that above the threshold level of $25,000 GNP per capita the levels and gradient in mortality are correlated with income inequality within societies. This threshold, he writes, 'represents a transition from the primacy of material constraints to social constraints as the limiting condition on the quality of human life' (Kawachi et al., 1999, p. 27).

However, while his main concern is what is happening above the threshold, Wilkinson may be far too quick in his conclusions about what is happening below the threshold. It is far from certain that determinants and distribution of premature mortality and impairments in societies under this threshold can be adequately explained as being due largely to material constraints, or lack of commodities such as healthcare. There may be a danger here again of confusing the cure with the cause. For example, the poor reproductive health of girls and women, including deplorable rates of maternal mortality, which are largely preventable, or the spread of HIV/AIDS are caused by social and cultural practices equally or more than material deprivations.

It would be even more misleading to conclude from Wilkinson's thesis of a transition from material to social constraints on quality of life that economic development in the form of rising GNP per capita will automatically bring with it improvements in life expectancy and lower prevalence of impairments. That is, by material constraints Wilkinson may be referring to broader material conditions than medical care to such things as food, water, sanitation, adequate shelter, clothing and so forth. There is a widely held view, particularly among economists, that economic growth inevitably leads to dramatic improvement in life expectancy, in infant mortality, decreases overall burden of impairments and improves social prosperity (Pritchett and

Summers, 1996; Bloom and Canning, 2007). It is a theory that is often attributed to Samuel Preston (Preston, 1975, 2007). And such a view underlies a theory of epidemiological transition describing the movement of societies from experiencing a high burden of infectious diseases to chronic diseases (Omran, 1971). However, Simon Szreter and others argue that there is little evidence from history of an automatic link between economic growth and improvement of health or welfare of individuals (Szreter, 1997; Biggs et al., 2010b).

In fact, Szreter, a historian of public health, argues that industrialization released very disruptive forces in British society that were managed by the politics of public-health advocates and institutions. That is, social action had an influential role in managing the process and consequences of industrialization which do not appear to be captured by Preston and Omran's theories. Sen also points to the modern-day importance of public discussion and agitation in the domain of health policy in such places as Thailand, India and China (Sen, 2011). In parallel discussions in economics, Sudhir Anand and Martin Ravillion show that indeed growth in GNP per capita is correlated with increasing life expectancy. But those improvements in life expectancies are largely explained by poverty alleviation programmes and spending on public health goods and services (Anand and Ravallion, 1993; Sen, 1999a). After accounting for these two factors, there is not much else left of the link between improvements in average incomes and life expectancy improvements. Biggs and colleagues have recently looked at twenty-two Latin American countries and shown that the relationship between GDP per capita and health is mediated by poverty levels and income inequality (Biggs et al., 2010a).

The point of dwelling on the relationship between economic development and health is the following. Both above and below the GNP per capita threshold, social factors determine health and longevity. The Wilkinson thesis draws attention primarily to incomes and then, reinforces the view that the health issues of rich countries are categorically different from those of poor countries; it is stated that social factors constrain the quality of life above while material factors constrain quality of life below. At the same time, the assertion is not that inequality in income above the threshold is directly causing poor health and other social problems. Instead, it is said that income inequality is measuring or reflecting how hierarchical a society is; it shows the scale of social differentiation and social distances within it (Wilkinson and Pickett, 2009, p. 27).

High levels of income inequality are produced by certain kinds of social arrangements that are corrosive as well as lead to further corrosive social arrangements. Wilkinson emphasizes that both processes impact the psychobiological pathways to disease in individuals during childhood as well as in adulthood. The distinction between social versus material factors on either side of the threshold seems to rely on the role of psychological factors related to relative social status influencing onset of disease above the threshold versus material affecting the health of individuals below the threshold. But why should Wilkinson consider psychosocial factors as the only social factors affecting health? As the research cited above by Szreter, Anand, Ravillion, Biggs and others shows, simple economic growth does not automatically improve health and longevity. These improve because of the implementation of certain kinds of social policies and arrangements, along with economic growth such as poverty alleviation and investments in medical and public health programmes. And, of course, there are the exemplary cases of Costa Rica, Cuba, Sri Lanka and the Indian state of Kerala, which achieve better health outcomes than many developed economies despite low GNP per capita (Sen, 1999a, pp. 46–47).

Social factors affect health and longevity below the threshold too; they can affect the availability and distribution of material goods as well as directly through psycho-social pathways. The threshold of when psychosocial factors related to relative inequality affect health should not be understood to mean that social factors do not affect health below it. Behind both the psychological pathways in richer countries and the material pathways in poorer countries are social factors. Emphasizing the threshold as being a tipping point from when material factors give way to socio-psycho-biological factors runs the risk of propagating the idea that rise in GNP automatically, or without any additional social policies, leads to improvements in health.

What is also worth noting is that Wilkinson and Pickett recommend a variety of interventions to reduce income inequality, including reducing gross income differences before taxes, and redistributive taxes and welfare programmes. Given their clear assertion that they are studying the phenomena of social hierarchy, it seems pretty clear that acting on incomes is really a means of reducing distances between social positions. Given that income inequality directly does not cause poor health – that is, the simple fact that one person's monthly wage is less than another person's wage does not induce disease in the former, it seems that our real focus is on what is happening in the lives of individuals. Intervening on incomes is only a means to helping individuals be able to avoid disease as well as other social deprivations. Across both rich and poor societies, and across all individuals, the relative influence of different kinds of factors on health will vary. In some places, health may be affected to a great extent through psychological pathways, while in other places it may be through material pathways determined by inadequate public spending on social goods. In both places we are interested in the individual's abilities to achieve various physical and mental functionings. So, acting on incomes to reduce income inequality can be one means in particular locations towards affecting the capabilities of individuals to achieve various physical and mental functionings. They surely are not the only means, and not necessarily the best means everywhere.

In light of the wide-ranging areas being researched by social epidemiologists to supplement the biomedical model, as well as the need to integrate debates on health and development that go beyond asserting simple causation between economic growth and health improvements, there is a need for what I immodestly term a 'unified theory' of health causation and distribution. Such a unified theory should be applicable across the entire human species and defensibly allocate responsibility for health causation and distribution among the four categories consisting of nature/biology, social conditions, environmental conditions, and individual behaviour/agency. I believe such a theory can indeed be developed by looking towards the 'entitlement analysis' used to explain the causes and distribution of acute and endemic malnutrition (famines). I review its history below and how it could be applied to health.

Entitlement analysis

Starting in the late 1970s, Jean Drèze and Amartya Sen sought to discredit or rather, demote a longstanding view influenced by Thomas Malthus that the cause of acute human starvation in developing countries is due to food scarcity, and more specifically, due to human populations outstripping the available food supply (Drèze and Sen, 1989). Such a view evolved and was substantiated by the observation at the individual level that starvation is caused by the lack of food and the study of natural laws such as predator–prey dynamics. In such a view, famine, disease and other widespread mortality are seen as natural checks on population growth. Drèze and Sen sought to undermine this view. They analysed data related to well-known historical cases of famines, and as economists often do, they built a model to try to explain the data. Their central finding was that the lack of food availability in an area was not an adequate general explanation or theory because mass starvation occurred where there was plenty of food, and starvation was avoided even where there was no food available locally. The existing explanatory model did not fit with the observable facts. They did not deny that every individual who starves did so because she did not have adequate nutrition. What they sought to show was that the availability or lack of availability of food in an area, in a population, was not a good indicator of whether people were starving, or their general nutritional status. One primary motivation for trying to show this is to help avoid the catastrophic consequences of public officials focusing on availability of grain or agricultural yields rather than looking directly at whether people are actually achieving suffi-cient nutrition. Their secondary conclusion was that most famines have been socially created either directly through particular social, economic, and political policies or from failures of government agen-cies to adequately respond.

Sen and Drèze were able to demonstrate how famines occur and their 'asymmetrical' effects on individuals by modelling the interac-tions between individuals and their external environment (Drèze and Sen, 1989). The exchange–entitlement analysis has three parts: endow-ments, exchange mechanisms and entitlement sets. The endowments include such things as physical assets, and of particular relevance are arable land, labour capacity and government transfers. Endowments include only legal sources and exclude assets acquired through means such as stealing or charitable organizations. Imagine that a person with a certain set of endowments stands in front of you on the left side. And, for most individuals, food sits in the market, which is in front of you. In the market, two kinds of exchanges are possible. The individual can exchange her labour or other assets such as crops, for money. And then, the individual makes a second exchange, with the money received from the first exchange, for food.

Drèze and Sen's unique and illuminating contribution to this basic descriptive market exchange model is that they also identified the concept of 'entitlement sets'. At any given point in time, a person who has certain endowments, such as labour capacity, can potentially exchange that endowment for certain wages which then can be poten-tially exchanged for a variety of bundles of goods, including food. The food then gets transformed by the individual into a certain level of being nourished. Therefore, an entitlement set consists of all the realistically possible bundles of goods that an individual can acquire through these two exchanges at a given time. It is similar to the notion in the world of finance called 'mark to market'; a product's value is determined by theoretically taking it to market to see what price it could fetch. At any given time, a person's entitlement set thus represents a 'mapping' starting from her initial endowments, moving through the two market mechanisms, to the possible different bundles of commodities, including goods for achieving nutrition. Moreover, such a mapping can be calculated theoretically, based on relevant information, without the individual's actually making either of the two exchanges. And, by measuring an entitlement set, it becomes possible to evaluate if the individual is capable of achieving adequate nutrition.

The central idea is that when an individual's entitlement set does not contain entitlements of sufficient bundles of food, because of a variety of factors implicated in the mapping, the person (or the family) will starve. Drawing on the data of the various periods of acute starvation, Drèze and Sen showed that starvation occurs not only when food is scarce, but also when food is plentiful because of a range of *social* factors operating through the two exchange mechanisms. For example, looking at the first exchange, when there is no work, or wages go down, individuals are not able to make exchanges for sufficient wages to then buy sufficient bundles of food. In the second exchange, when prices of food go up because food is being exported out or being hoarded locally, individuals may not be able to acquire sufficient bundles of food. Background institutional or social factors and the independent and interactive dynamics of both exchange mechanisms determine whether individuals are realistically able to acquire sufficient bundles of food for becoming adequately nourished.

At the same time, the kinds and levels of *endowments* that an individual has also impact the sufficiency of food entitlements. When individuals do not have any assets such as arable land (e.g. landless peasants) they become extremely vulnerable to factors affecting wages and food prices while striving to achieve sufficient nutrition. Disabled individuals or those restricted from working outside the home are constrained in their abilities to exchange labour for wages, and those wages for food bundles. Moreover, where an individual has extra-nutritional needs because she is growing, is pregnant, or breastfeeding, she may be more susceptible to malnutrition because her entitlement set does not expand in tandem with her changing biological needs. An individual's unique biological *needs* and *agency* or abilities to engage with or transform external conditions thus, also affect the breadth of her entitlement set. Because it parses out the causation of malnutrition into different factors, one profound insight of this model is that it reveals how social policies aiming to treat citizens equally by which they ration an equal or standard amount of food to every individual would be blind to – or exhibit indifference to – the possible malnutrition of individuals who have extra nutritional needs or agency constraints. The differences in endowments, particularly physical and mental endowments as well as agency skills significantly affect the size of the entitlement sets they can produce as well as the size of the entitlement sets they need to achieve the same level of functioning as others.

By building an analytical model of the causation of malnutrition that identifies the role of personal endowments and needs, individual agency, social conditions such as market-exchange mechanisms, and physical conditions (food availability), Drèze and Sen were able to produce more comprehensive explanations of malnutrition than those which focused on food scarcity. Their model is more robust than the food scarcity model because it is able to explain the causation and distribution of malnutrition, even when food supply is plentiful, and no matter the time or place. Importantly, the model's conceptual framework is able to provide analysis of acute starvation as well as endemic malnutrition during non-famine periods. An individual's experience of low-level malnutrition is determined by the same range of factors as during periods of acute starvation: her biological endowments/needs, agency skills, factors affecting the two market-exchange mechanisms, and physical availability of food. Because the exchange-entitlement model has such broad explanatory power, it has now come to be viewed as the *general theory* of malnutrition with enormous influence on food policy.

It is of paramount importance to Sen to point out that focusing on the availability of food would probably lead to the non-recognition of wide-scale malnutrition or starvation. Measuring food availability per-capita, crop-yields, or levels of grain-stores would be the wrong place to look to measure or prevent acute starvation and low-level malnutrition. Instead, focusing on individual entitlement sets and their sufficiency for achieving adequate nutrition for that individual would more accurately reflect the risk and prevalence of malnutrition in times of acute crisis or otherwise. While this simple model may seem to involve only the individual and the market, Sen and Drèze are emphatic that both the public and the government can play significant roles in ensuring that the entitlement sets of individuals contain sufficient food during famines, and in addressing endemic hunger. Their model is also able to show that starvation was avoided or alleviated even where there was no food available because social factors such as a free press and community agitation compelled a government response.

The power of the exchange–entitlement analysis lies not only in its robust explanations of malnutrition, but also in its potential application to broader health issues and indeed, to all quality of life issues.

Sen's argument against focusing on food availability is the same one used against focusing on GDP as the primary focus of economic development policy as well as for rejecting the focus on resources in social justice theories. And we can apply the same reasoning to identify the deficiency in focusing on how much a society spends on healthcare. Instead, we should be interested in the 'health entitlement sets' of individuals or, as the present book argues, their capabilities of being healthy.

The move from the entitlement theory to capability theory, and then to health capability should not be very hard to understand. The entitlement analysis identifies the causation and differing distribution of malnutrition across individuals by looking at the interactions between an individual's endowments and exchange mechanisms. The entitlement set represents all the potential bundles of goods one could acquire, and one assesses if these bundles could be sufficient to meet nutritional needs. In comparison a person's capability set consists of 'beings and doings' such as being adequately nourished. The capability to be adequately nourished is then not just determined by the availability of food, but also by the nature of exchange mechanisms and personal features or endowments. Capability theory posits that personal features plus social conditions (inclusive of material conditions) and environmental conditions result in a capability.

Diversity in personal features – the diversity in needs and skills to convert social conditions and material goods – and the actual social and physical conditions determine the content of the capability set. In the CA, the endowments in famine analysis is transformed into purely personal biological and mental features, their internal biological endowments, needs, and skills. And the market exchanges component is transformed into broader material and social conditions.

To be even more explicit, the CA can be easily summarized as individual needs and skills (endowments) plus social conditions (two-step market exchange dynamics plus commodities) and physical conditions produce capabilities. The capability theory is simply the broadening out of the entitlement theory as the capability set contains bundles of all human 'beings and doings', and not just possible goods acquired from the market.

Famines and epidemiology

The analysis of famines and malnutrition is amenable to being transposed onto a theory of health causation and distribution, not least because the framework successfully explains malnutrition, an obvious health concern. Drawing on Drèze and Sen's analysis, an individual's 'health entitlements' or 'CH entitlement set' would contain the potential beings and doings produced from the interactions of: (1) individual biological needs; (2) abilities to convert material and social conditions into health functionings; (3) the extant social conditions; and (4) the environmental conditions. Failure to achieve such functionings as living a normal length of lifespan or avoiding impairments can be causally explained by the independent and interactive effects of all these factors. We must keep in mind, however, that social conditions still have greater reach than other factors and operate directly at the individual level and at the supra-individual level. That is, referring back to the famines example, social factors can cause a specific individual not to acquire enough bundles of food to be sufficiently nourished as well as shape the market-exchange mechanisms, agrarian policies, commodities trading and emergency food programmes.

The descriptive model of entitlement sets or capabilities allows for the integration of the biomedical model of disease causation as well as the diverse range of social determinant theories of causation and distribution. At bottom, both epidemiology and economics rely on statistical analysis to infer causation from correlation. The capability model, which comes out of economics, has no difficulty in being able to analyse objective features such as biological functionings and material goods or qualitative phenomena such as conversion skills and social conditions. Thus, individual-level biomedical causes such as genetic endowments, exposures to harmful substances, and behaviours can be integrated with the analysis of social determinant causes such as workplace conditions, social support, political and economic policies, and so forth.

Indeed, the capabilities framework can integrate all of the various social determinants models. It is clear that across individuals and groups, the influence of different personal endowments, conversion skills and exposures to material goods and social conditions cause different and asymmetric health constraints. Importantly, the capability model provides the significant conceptual advantage of viewing health as a possible set of functionings rather than as the absence of disease. Using the concept of health as capability to achieve or exercise a set of capabilities and functionings would allow this explanatory model to be applicable across the human species, and across rich and poor countries.

The further advantage of the capability model is that it is conducive to undertaking an ethical analysis of what the social response should be to the causation and distribution of health constraints. The biomedical model and the social determinants models are constrained from providing valuable ethical information. For example, social determinants research has been motivated by and in turn, expanded social concern for the unequal social distribution of health constraints. However, the scope of social epidemiologists' concern is still only limited to social distributions that are causally linked to social determinants. For example, skewed mortality rates across social classes may be attributed to various psychological stressors due to class position. But cutting across social classes, there may also be unequal mortality across ethnic groups. Though members of the ethnic group may belong to many classes with different mortality rates, there still may be a compelling reason to address absolute and unequal mortality within the ethnic group in addition to addressing unequal mortality rates across classes. The consequences may be greater for members of the ethnic group, or there may be a social commitment to especially protect the group from premature mortality. Even if there is no social cause to the distribution, there may still be good reason to identify patterns of distributions according to social markers. The biomedical model and even the social determinants model can only legitimately examine distribution patterns according to causal factors.

In contrast, the capability framework can identify distribution patterns of capability sets across multiple dimensions of individuals and groups. This can provide valuable information in determining the response to the causes, distributions and consequences of health capability and its constraints. Health, understood as the ability to achieve vital goals or a cluster of capabilities and functionings, provides the standard against which to compare a particular individual's health capability set. The capability causation framework provides much richer information on different possible causes of constraints on the achievement of the cluster of capabilities that make up health.

Moreover, social responses to the health capability sets of a single individual or group when they fall below the standard requires looking at differences in causes (endowments, skills, physical and social conditions, choices) as well as asymmetric distributions, and consequences. In the simple case where the cause is the same, looking at a variety of distribution patterns across social groupings or according to consequences may be necessary to prioritize social responses. In contrast to such analysis being on the margins of classic or social epidemiology, the unified capability theory of health causation and distribution can provide robust descriptive information on causation and distribution that can inform an effective and ethical social response.

Malthusian thesis and the biomedical model

The detailed discussion on the exchange–entitlement analysis hope-fully makes it easier to see the bases of the affinity between social epidemiology and capabilities approach. Drèze and Sen's investigation into famine data and modelling of the causation and distribution of malnutrition has remarkable similarities with contemporary social epidemiology. To wit, social epidemiology also strives to explain the causation and distribution of ill-health. The deficiency of the individual-level 'bio-medical' model is that it is unable to explain adequately the causation of many chronic diseases as well as their social distribution patterns. Therefore, social epidemiologists also aim to demote the predominant explanatory paradigm in epidemiology that disease is caused by factors including genetic endowment, volitional behaviours and exposures to harmful particles. They have expanded the scope of the causal chain and causal factors by identifying the social factors affecting the three proximate causes as well as identifying new socio-psycho-biological pathways to disease. In Sen's analyses of famines and social epidemiology the severe deficiencies in the dominant explanatory model's abilities fully to explain phenomena motivates a broadening the scope of causal factors and the search for a better explanatory model. However, that is not all they share in common.

The role of nature is also contested in both analyses. Drèze and Sen shifted the burden of responsibility for acute starvation from natural phenomenon to social conditions. Social epidemiologists are trying for the same. Marmot, for example, aims to show that the social gradient in health achievements across all societies is not a purely natural phenomenon or sufficiently explained by the focus on individual-level factors. The steepness of the gradient – the extent of health inequality – is also shown to be affected by social policies. Moreover, Sen was focused on criticizing the narrow focus on food scarcity and pursued identifying the important role of personal features and social conditions. Social epidemiologists have less to achieve in some respects, as epidemiology already accepts the influence of biology, behaviour and material conditions. The insights and controversy are with respect to the direct influence of social conditions.

Both frameworks seek to build an explanatory causal model that integrates the factors of personal features, agency, and material and social conditions. Sen's two exchange mechanisms have their counter-parts in the analysis of ill-health. It may be easy to begin with the exchange for the commodity of healthcare; from there, to the concept of epidemiological exchanges between individuals. However, social epidemiology expands the idea of exchange to encompass the discreet, continuous, or reiterative social exchanges made between individuals and their environment over the life course. The important difference between the two is that social epidemiology has not identified anything like the entitlement set. However, the great similarities and overlap between the two frameworks suggest that there is good reason to begin conceptualizing human health as health-entitlement sets and even, as a capability to be healthy.

Conclusion

To summarize the previous two chapters of Part I, the argument illustrated how coherence could be brought to the concept of health in the theory and practice of the health sciences through a concept of health as the capability to achieve a vital or basic cluster of capabilities and functionings. It also put forward a theory of causation and distribution of health that is able to account for individual-level, proximate causes as well as social determinants. Such a theory unifies a broad range of dichotomous frameworks such those used to evaluate infectious versus chronic diseases, biomedical versus social determinants, rich versus poor country health profiles, proximate versus distal causative agents, natural versus social science, individual versus social levels and so forth. Moreover, the framework also provides rich information for identifying an ethical social response to the inequalities in health by looking at the inequalities in health capabilities – at the different aspects of causal components, social distribution patterns, consequences, persistence, and possibilities of social remedies.

Part II

3

The Capabilities Approach

The aim of this chapter is to present a brief overview of the capabilities approach (CA) in order to situate the argument for the capability to be healthy (CH) in the next chapter. I outline some key insights of the CA and some of the major differences with other theoretical approaches to social justice. I will end with some key criticisms made against the CA and highlight some live issues at the frontier of the theory with an eye towards those issues especially relevant to the CH. Throughout the discussion I also point out some of the main differences between the approaches of Amartya Sen and Martha Nussbaum but I do not review the small but growing number of other variants of the CA.[1] Indeed, the CH argument I am advancing can be understood to be a hybrid argument which integrates Sen's 'analytical device' of capability and emphasis on freedoms with Nussbaum's central human capabilities as the content. Just to explain this hybridity a bit further, the CH is presented in Chapter 4 as a meta-capability to achieve a cluster of central human capabilities and functionings each at a threshold level that is commensurate with equal dignity worthy of the human being living in the contemporary world.

I shall be arguing that the CH is a kind of freedom which is intrinsically and instrumentally valuable, which is a profoundly Senian concern. And the CH is also grounded in dignity and equal respect which is distinct to Nussbaum's reasoning about capabilities. The discussion of the CA in this chapter aims to provide the background to developing and fleshing out such a hybrid argument. Given the increasing breadth and seemingly exponential rise in the quantity of academic publications on the CA, my intention here is modest, as I only present a focused summary. Needless to say, a synopsis or sketch of something that is seen to be a broad intellectual movement, and which has at least two prominent versions, will not be a satisfactory account in many aspects. Nevertheless, I present what I believe are some salient aspects of the CA.

The origins of the 'capability' or 'capabilities' approach lie in the critique of the thinking and prevailing paradigms in development economics and policy as well as moral and political philosophy in the 1970s and 1980s. More specifically, the focus on capabilities was initially theorized by Amartya Sen. It was borne out of his analysis of famines as well as from his reflections on Kenneth Arrow's *Social Choice and Individual Values* and John Rawls' arguments that were eventually published as *A Theory of Justice* (Arrow, 1951; Rawls, 1971; Sen, 1976, 1977, 1981b, 1981a; Drèze and Sen, 1989).[2] The first public articulation of the CA in the domain of political philosophy is usually identified as being Sen's 1979 Tanner Lecture on Human Values titled 'Equality of What?' (Sen, 1982b). In that lecture, Sen proposed that the concern for justice and equality should not be in the space of subjective mental welfare, resources, or negative liberties but in the space of human capabilities, what individuals are realistically able to be and do in their lives. Since that lecture the CA has been profoundly transforming the theory and practice of a wide range of academic disciplines including development studies, welfare economics, social policy, political philosophy, political science, public health, education and even engineering. It has also influenced public policy in various areas. For instance, the CA is evident in the greater attention given to inequality or distributional concerns by international development organizations, in the World Bank's Voices of the Poor project,[3] as the basis for the UN Human Development Index and human development reports,[4] in the background research papers for the United Kingdom's National Equalities Commission,[5] as the basis of the second and third national reports on poverty and wealth in Germany,[6] in the national strategy for public health in Sweden,[7] and most recently in Sarkozy's Commission on the Measurement of Economic Performance and Social Progress,[8] The broad influence of the CA on a wide variety of academic disciplines, on the theoretical underpinnings or justification of policies, and directly on the content of policies themselves lends to seeing it as both an intellectual movement and programme for action. It is a set of ideas that questions, clarifies, disputes, and presents an alternative to some dominant ideas or the status quo affecting the well-being of individuals and societies. As such, it is also seen as a revolutionary 'counter theory'.

The CA particularly targets theories and policies that focus on commodities such as incomes or on subjective mental welfare, as well as policies that aim for maximization without adequate concern for distribution or equity. The focus on capabilities and equity is at the core of the CA. While capabilities are said to be a more coherent focus of justice, equity or equality is also seen to be a central part of a conception of justice. According to Sen, there is nothing logical about the link between equality and justice, but that no theory of justice would be plausible in modern society that does not treat all individuals equally (Sen, 1996b). Sen, Nussbaum, and others have written numerous books and academic analyses on the CA. And much of the literature is well documented in the online bibliography of The Human Development and Capability Association.[9]

Commodities off-target

The CA is an analytical and ethical framework which asserts that societies should focus on supporting – nurturing, protecting, providing, expanding, restoring, and so forth – the capabilities of individuals to conceive, pursue, and revise their life plans (Sen, 1999a; Alkire, 2002, 2005b; Robeyns, 2005a; Nussbaum, 2006; Vizard, 2006). This is often stated in the CA literature as helping people 'be and do what they have reason to value'. The focus on capabilities to be and doing things is initially motivated by the recognition that economic goods such as income and material wealth or commodities only have instrumental value for what individuals are able to be or do through using or 'converting' such goods. Therefore, instead of focusing on goods because of their instrumental value, CA advocates contend that we should target our reasoning about social justice and social policy directly on what we really care about namely, what individuals are able to be and do in their lives. The space between commodities and what people can actually do in their lives, while often erased by many theorists by conflating the two things, is given much attention by the CA. I discuss this more below.

The language of capabilities refers to the real practical possibility of an individual being able to be and do certain things while 'functionings' refer to the achieved outcomes. A capability is also seen as having a real opportunity. And, as I have been arguing in this book, a human capability can be broken down into the causal components of individual endowments and needs, external physical and social conditions, and individual behaviour or agency. A person's capability to be or doing something is determined by the independent or interactive causal roles of all these four factors. And to be clear, CA advocates do not deny that economic or other physical goods can be critically important or valuable for individuals. Things such as income, food, medical care or adequate shelter can be life-saving, and it would be wholly misguided to deny that. Rather, they are asserting that an exclusive or primary focus on goods or instrumental means rather than on what individuals are able to be and do with those goods is off-target; it appears to be 'fetishistic' and produces various kinds of informational and moral errors with unacceptable consequences.

The consequence of theoretical deliberations or practical policies being off-target by focusing on commodities is that the theory or policy can lead to neglecting, tolerating, or exacerbating inequalities in what individuals are able to be and do; the things that make up their quality of life, well-being and freedoms. Sen states this point simply as a misconceived theory can kill (Sen, 1999a, p. 209). Focusing on 'things' obscures what we really care about as well as hinders recognizing the possible inequalities in what people are actually able to be and do in their lives. In the first instance, the CA argues that it is incorrect to conclude from seeing that people have things or that there are things available in the environment, that people are able to use these goods as effectively as others in order to pursue their life plans. Instead, the CA motivates us actually to look at what individuals are able to be and do in their lives. Referring back to the famine analysis in the previous chapter, as the data showed, it is not reliable to think that food availability reflects the nutritional achievements of individuals. Various kinds of barriers, all perfectly legal, could be preventing individuals from achieving adequate nutrition. Abstracting from that, one should not conclude that the availability of goods, including income, indicates that individuals are doing well in their lives.

One of the rejoinders to this argument for focusing on capabilities rather than on goods or 'resources' is that there is actually not that much difference between focusing on resources or capabilities. Because the goods are valued for creating opportunities for people to pursue their life plans, and the amounts of goods can be distributed according to need by including some additional information, a 'sophisticated resource theory' does as much as an approach that focuses on capabilities (Pogge, 2002a, 2010). This debate becomes more complicated in academic philosophy where goods or resources are not just physical things but include ethical social goods such as liberties, opportunities or social bases of self-respect.

Sen made his criticism against physical resources as well as these social goods. In any case, the argument against capabilities goes that focusing on these things is not so off base and offers various advantages such as allowing for public transparency, measurability, and efficient ranking or prioritization. These are virtues that the CA is seen to lack. There is also a possible philosophical move whereby what people are able to be and do are themselves categorized as 'personal resources' or individual resource holdings (Dworkin, 2000, pp. 299–303; Williams, 2002; Pierik and Robeyns, 2007). This move, then, seems to erase the distinction between resources and capabilities. I will not go further into these debates or try to resolve them here.

Persistent inequalities

If the first motivating concern is to point out the mistake in looking at commodity holdings a second, foundational and motivating impetus behind the CA is the 'real-world' concern for persistent inequalities in the quality of life of individuals and finding extant measures or goals of development and social progress lacking in capturing the moral concern for such inequalities. Though it is related to the first point about the focus on goods being off-target, this concern expresses the worry that national or aggregate group statistics such as Gross National Product (GNP) or averages such as GNP per capita and population average health statistics often obfuscate great inter-individual inequalities in basic human functionings as well as in broader opportunities and abilities to pursue life plans. The familiar focus on aggregate measurements of achievements of national populations such as GNP probably reflect societal goals of maximizing the total or average group levels of wealth or welfare; what you measure is often what you end up aiming to achieve. The CA militates against both a narrow focus on material goods such as incomes or aggregate GNP as well as against maximizing aggregate indicators while disregarding inter-individual inequalities in what individuals are actually able to be and do.[10] Instead, the CA champions supporting every individual's capabilities, understood as freedoms or real opportunities to achieve beings and doings.

At the same time, advocates of the CA have different views about when the goal of social action is to ensure the sufficiency, equity, absolute equality or some other level of capabilities. They also disagree on which capabilities societies should be guaranteed, even initially. Nussbaum has been arguing that every human being should have social support to achieve ten particular capabilities, each at certain sufficient thresholds.[11] Others argue for a core set of capabilities necessary for political equality, some for 'shortfall equity' in some capabilities, and still others argue that the choice of capabilities and their levels will be and should be determined by 'partial orderings' as reasoning about justice can involve incommensurable values both internally as well as externally across individuals. Furthermore, Sen has gone to great lengths to state that he does not support a single or pre-defined rule about the kinds or levels of capabilities. Instead, he advocates taking a comparative and contextual approach to each situation in order to determine the capability and its distribution across individuals.

As a result of the differing approaches to inequalities in capabilities, some authors have asked whether once it is decided that individual capabilities are the right focus, would the CA support maximization of capabilities? If capabilities are the right focus of our moral concern, should we not aim to maximize capabilities? If not, does that mean the CA would sacrifice improving the capabilities of the many for the sake of improving the capabilities of the few? Many CA advocates seemingly avoid this and other questions regarding aggregation issues. Nussbaum has the clearest answer which is that ensuring sufficiency of capabilities has priority over maximizing the total or average capabilities of a population. But this leads to a problem identified by Peter Singer as well as Richard Arneson. They both ask Nussbaum what she would do in a situation where the effort and resources needed to bring one individual above the sufficiency threshold could alternatively be used to expand the capabilities of many individuals (Singer, 2002).

Consider one scenario where everyone is below the sufficiency threshold and the choice is between helping to get one person to the sufficiency threshold, versus those of two or more closer to the threshold. A theory that espouses a right to sufficient capabilities seems to give no guidance on how to deal with the rights of many individuals. In a second scenario, there is a choice between spending enormous resources to improve one individual's capabilities just a little bit more in order to get them to sufficiency while everyone else is above the threshold and the resources could improve their capabilities quite substantially. Not helping the larger number, even if it increases equality, looks as though it is equalizing down the capabilities of the many;

and does it matter if the single individual is improving only by a little bit to get to sufficiency or by a lot? This simple case, referred to as the 'aggregation problem' or 'resource monster problem' can be presented in many different variations. While the CA may have substantive arguments for focusing on capabilities, it does not at present offer any clear solutions to these kinds of distributional problems. It is clear that for there to be meaningful application of the CA, such problems have to be tackled head on. Nussbaum would argue, drawing on Hegel, these clashes of right with right are tragic cases that challenge us first to think about how such situations have arisen and design a future where such clashes would not arise (Nussbaum, 2000a, p. 127). And Sen would probably address distributional problems through public reasoning aimed at partial orderings of outcomes.

My own view is that such scenarios require evaluation across the dimensions of causes, levels, persistence, consequences and possible responses. Such thought experiments, by isolating consideration of only one of these dimensions, force us to make moral errors. That is, forcing a trade-off between spending social resources on the one versus the many excludes the possibility that justice demands that the resources be spent on the one because of the types of causes of her impairments, the consequences she will experience, or the type of social intervention that is needed for her versus that for the others. The CA motivates looking at aggregation problems much more as multi-dimensional problems than largely as trade-offs between the interests of the few versus the many. I leave for now the queston of whether these responses to aggregation problems are adequate or coherent.

Recognizing diversity

Continuing with the CA's critique of the focus on resources, CA advocates also identify that the methods used in identifying and distributing resources can actually create or exacerbate inequalities in the choices and abilities of individuals. In both theory and policy-making, the types and amounts of resources to be distributed are often based on a standard or idealized conception of individual/citizens or their needs. An institution might ask how much monthly income an 'average person' needs to pay for 'basic requirements'. Consequently, that amount of income is provided to all individuals irrespective of what their particular needs might be. However, at any single point in time, and over the life course, every human being differs in her biological and psychological needs for the types and quantities of material goods, social conditions and physical environments in order to achieve the same level of functioning as another human being.

For example, a pregnant woman needs more iron and nutrition than another individual who is not pregnant, in order to undertake the same level of physical activity. Or, the daily requirements for protein are greater for a growing child than an older individual on any given day. Or, simply, a person with higher metabolism may need more nutritional intake. Distributing one standard package of goods, such as a minimum income or food rations, based either on a fixed conception of a person including their needs or capacities, will result in the individuals who receive those goods becoming unequally able to achieve the same functionings, as well as their individually diverse plans of life. Human beings are inherently diverse, and such diversity has to be recognized when trying to theorize or implement policies affecting their well-being.

Endowments and needs

The relevance of diversity in needs is not just a concern about commodities or about poor individuals getting government rations or welfare benefits; it could apply as easily to wealthy individuals in wealthy countries. For example, a pregnant woman in a wealthy country may need different working arrangements from those of a non-pregnant woman or a man. But if the working arrangements are designed around someone who is not or cannot be pregnant, the needs of the pregnant woman may go unsatisfied or be seen to be extraordinary needs. And this may be how the diverse needs of other individuals come to be seen when a theory or policy is based on a standard template. Moreover, such situations, where some individuals end up having more choices than others, or some individuals become able to do a particular thing better than others, not only can leave the needs of some individuals unsatisfied or exacerbate their deprivation, it can also affect their sense of self respect; the situation may induce feelings of shame for not 'fitting the mould' as well as for not being of equal standing with others. Whether it is the size of welfare benefits, the type and shape of the entrance to a building, or entitlements in ethical theory, using a standard conception of individuals that ignores the inherent diversity in the endowments and needs of human beings at any given point in time or over the life course will create or exacerbate inequalities in what individuals can do and be in their lives.

Conversion skills

Every individual also differs in her abilities to 'convert' income and commodities as well as her surrounding physical and social conditions into beings and doings. These abilities to convert things and conditions can be due to internal or external factors. For example, physical and psychological features such as having a disability or being illiterate can profoundly determine one's ability to make use of available material goods and social conditions. And no matter how internally capable an individual might be, the external physical and social conditions can significantly impact if and how well an individual can practically achieve beings and doings. For example, racism, gender, and caste discrimination, or disabling architecture are some obvious significant barriers to an individual being able to convert extant goods and social conditions into beings and doings.[12] Individuals can also be differently able to convert their own endowments – their own physical features, reasoning capacity, or even property – because of the lack of information, training, and indeed, various types of cultural beliefs or social practices.

For example, in a social environment where knowledge about sex and reproduction is considered to be morally suspect, the lack of information may lead girls and women to believe that certain kinds of reproductive tract impairments are a normal part of being female. In other cultures, including developed countries, girls and women many believe that females cannot physically exert themselves as much as males, or that reasoning skills of females are ill-equipped for business or scientific professions. And lastly, an extension to the point made earlier about diversity in needs is that individuals may be unable to convert their own endowments, such as physical features or reasoning skills, because they are mentally or physically severely impaired. In such cases, the social conditions, including the conditions affecting their carers, exert a profound influence on what such individuals are able to be and do in their lives.

So, aside from diversity in internal needs and characteristics, individuals differ in abilities to transform external physical and social conditions and their own endowments into beings and doings that constitute their daily living. Sen identifies four external 'conversion factors' that affect individuals differently aside from their differences in internal factors. These include (i) diversities in physical environment, (ii) variations in social climate, (iii) differences in relational perspectives, and (iv) distribution within the family (Sen, 1999a, pp. 70–71, 2009, pp. 255–256). These conversion factors also form the basis of the causal model of capability I advocate in this book. I will not go into further detail here about these factors but present them in order to show that the CA is centrally concerned with and engages in detailed analysis about the diversity in the needs and conversion skills of individuals and how these affect their absolute and relative capabilities of pursuing beings and doings. And by doing so, the CA asserts the moral relevance of recognizing the diversity of individuals and criticizes the use of a standard conception or template of individuals and their needs, the effects of external factors affecting their conversion skills, or simply ignoring needs and conversion skills all together. Not recognizing the inherent diversity in needs and the conversion factors that affect every human being will result in tolerating or exacerbating inequalities in quality of life across individuals.

Welfare

Given the CA's central worries over the right target of ethical concern and inequalities in the quality of life of individuals, the CA also strongly rejects the prevalent focus on subjective welfare – whether it is utility, happiness, preferences, or satisfaction. This focus on welfare is found in moral and political philosophy and economics. Consequently, the focus on mental welfare is also present in national and international economic and development policies. The pervasive focus in economics on welfare or utility is due to the influence of the philosophy of utilitarianism. In fact, the most important early English economists before 1900 were also the most prominent utilitarian philosophers (Rawls and Freeman, 2007, p. 162). Paralleling utilitarian philosophy, which asserts that the only correct or justifiable social goal is to maximize human happiness and minimize pain across individuals, welfare economics aims to maximize the social welfare function that aggregates preferences.

However, as has been repeatedly argued by numerous authors, welfare economics suffers from certain limitations because the underlying utility maximization philosophy is seen to be deficient. At least three major faults of utilitarianism have been historically identified. The philosophy does not care that preferences are malleable; it is indifferent to inequalities; and it does not respect some basic rights or other important values (Sen and Williams, 1982; Nussbaum, 2000b).

To explain further, some human beings adapt to great deprivation and express little or no dissatisfaction. Meanwhile, other individuals can express great dissatisfaction with what objectively is a minor annoyance in comparison. If much greater aggregate welfare would be created from addressing the minor needs of the most intense complainers, then that takes priority over addressing absolute or relative deprivations. While intensity is one issue, it is also possible that addressing a minor problem of a great many like a headache can create more aggregate welfare than a significant problem of one individual, such as one who is suffering from AIDS. So utilitarianism is welfarist in that it values only subjective well-being, whether a person is happy or satisfied, and it is rigidly consequentialist in that the right action to pursue is seen only in the outcomes and will maximize subjective well-being. It is also seen to require rigidly full or complete rank-ordering of every option.

Moreover, under a pure utilitarian regime, the goal of maximizing aggregate welfare as the ultimate principle of justice means that it is reasonable for any individual human being to be used as a means of achieving higher aggregate social welfare. The feeding of Christians to the lions in the Roman coliseum for the entertainment of the masses would be acceptable and indeed required as it creates more utility than not do so. It is a philosophy that does not recognize or respect the inviolability of every human being. Aside from this fundamental weakness, there is also the issue of the primacy given to the pursuit of happiness by utilitarianism. Certain actions may be important to pursue, even though they are known to result in unhappiness. Fighting in a just revolution, or saving someone from drowning can be valuable activities even though they will be unlikely to bring pleasure or happiness to the individual. Though this cursory description of utilitarianism may be criticized as being an unfair thumbnail sketch, it does, however, identify the types of reasons that critics of utilitarianism have used to argue that deliberations on social justice, equity and economic and social policies must consist of much more than just maximizing subjective preferences, pleasure or satisfaction.[13]

Capabilities not commodities or welfare

To avoid what are seen to be profound flaws in both the theory and policy implementation of 'resourcist' and 'welfarist' approaches, advocates of the CA aver that the equal respect for the moral worth of every human being compels the ensuring of sufficient and equitable capabilities of individuals to conceive and pursue their life plans. Furthermore, in a liberal society, the state should aim to secure people's capabilities and not functionings, except in cases such as those of children and severely disabled adults, because there is intrinsic value in having free choice to determine one's life plans. Moreover, a state directly inducing people's functionings may endorse and elevate a certain kind of human life over others, violating the requirement of state neutrality about competing conceptions of the good life.[14] Citizens must be allowed to determine their own life plans as far as possible.

The CA also gives much attention to the important distinction between 'substantive' opportunity and just formal opportunity. Substantive freedom or opportunity exists when there is a real or effective practical possibility of exercising a capability. That is, for each capability, a person's internal features/needs and conversion skills and external physical and social conditions all must match sufficiently in such a way as to create the practical possibility for the person to achieve the being or doing. CA advocates also emphasize the value of having a meaningful breadth of capabilities.[15] That is, the intent of the CA can be undermined if the idea of a capability is applied to superfluous or harmful beings and doings, or a person is presented with a very limited choice of capabilities, even if they are valuable.

Because of Sen's background in development economics, the CA for the first decade or so was viewed as being most directly relevant to the theory and practice of economic and social development policies of developing countries. Given that alleviating poverty and human deprivation is the main concern of such policy arenas, and that prevailing policies focused largely on increasing aggregate wealth or distributing basic goods, the CA was viewed as offering the latest or most state-of-the-art policy guidance that can overcome the drawbacks of previous policies, while also providing more coherent ethical justification. That view still remains.

However, the social concern over poverty, inequality and other deprivations in industrialized countries also means that the CA has potential for global application. Indeed, its influence is now also increasingly becoming visible in the public deliberations and policies in high-income countries. For example, in European countries the CA is being applied in a variety of domains including economic policies,[16] social equality policies,[17] health reviews,[18] and even political party manifestos.[19] However, what is becoming more widely recognized is that while the CA initially had significant interest and influence in development economics and policy, Sen was engaged as intensely and directly with many of the most prominent moral and political philosophers and their theories since the late 1970s.

Rawls, Sen and Nussbaum

Much of modern-day egalitarianism has its roots in the eighteenth and nineteenth centuries, when utilitarianism presented a radically alternative ethical framework to counteract longstanding social inequalities arising from such arbitrary events as the class and family one was born into or from pursuing one's religious beliefs. Utilitarians shed the pretences of the state of nature and natural laws and, instead, advocated the moral importance of 'utility' and taking equal account of the welfare of every individual in social planning. It found wide acceptance due to its simple method of consequentialist reasoning, which was simply to achieve welfare maximization. Its justification being that welfare or happiness is the most important good in every human life; what is at the most fundamental base of individual actions. Utilitarianism and its single prescription to achieve 'the greatest good' continues to dominate public policy-making in countries world-wide and operates as a tacit background for contemporary deliberations about social justice.

After dominating liberal political and social philosophy for over a century, the philosophy of utilitarianism was seriously challenged in the late twentieth century, most of all by the publication in 1971 of *A Theory of Justice* by John Rawls (Rawls, 1971). Rather than simply providing additional criticisms, Rawls offered an alternative theory. Resurrecting the social contract tradition, Rawls proposed that in a hypothetical decision-making process, a representative group of human beings, placed behind a 'veil of ignorance' that shields them from knowledge of their prospective social positions would impartially identify a set of basic social institutions, entitlements and rules for distributing these entitlements, which then would constitute the basic structure of a just or well-ordered society. This conception of social justice is argued to exemplify a 'fair procedure' approach to justice as it identifies a mutually agreed, fair process for decision-making so that the outcomes, whatever they might turn out to be, will be considered just (Nussbaum, 2006, p. 10). This is in contrast to alternative approaches including utilitarianism or rights theories which seek to ensure certain outcomes, and then proceed to identify appropriate procedures (Nussbaum, 2006, pp. 81–84). Rawls made changes to his theory but what I discuss here are aspects that remained constant.

According to Rawls the respect for the equal moral worth of persons is expressed in his theory in a variety of ways – in the hypothetical procedure and, most particularly, in the social guarantee of a set of 'primary goods'.[20] That is, respect for the equal moral worth of individuals is partly realized through ensuring that every individual has access to certain goods which every rational individual would find to be instrumentally valuable in pursuing their individually unique ends. The primary goods are 'all purpose means' that include material goods such as income and wealth, as well as social conditions such as liberties, equality of opportunity to achieve jobs and offices, and social basis for self-respect. These are all seen to be resources because they are goods that are socially created and distributed.

Rawls further maintained that against the background of a set of basic institutions which would guarantee the highest equal basic liberties and then equality of opportunity, certain inequalities in income and wealth should be allowed. Rawls reasoned that equalizing incomes would take away incentives for individuals which are necessary for the economy to function and grow. Inequalities in income and wealth were unavoidable in order for economic growth, but they could be regulated or harnessed. Thus, Rawls stipulated that keeping in mind the requirement for the priority and equal distribution of certain primary goods (such as liberty, or social bases of self-respect), any increase in inequality in income and wealth across individuals could be allowed if it also increased the shares of the least well-off as much as possible.

The significance of Rawls' contributions to moral and political philosophy is hard to overstate. He is credited with single-handedly re-invigorating political philosophy. Other philosophers have followed Rawls in offering alternative conceptions of social justice and, given his influence in the field, have had to articulate the similarities and differences to his theory and also to utilitarianism to some extent.

After surveying the field of political philosophy including and after Rawls, Sen makes the observation that all the proposed modern theories of social justice are egalitarian or give equality a central place, but the central and divisive question is: equality of what? (Sen, 1992a). Sen argues that in order for a conception of social justice to be plausible in the modern world, every individual has to be treated equally; but in what respect should individuals be treated equally? Rawls conceives the moral equality of persons as requiring a particular distribution of particular primary goods. Contemporary utilitarians still maintain that equality requires taking into account each person's utility in the maximization of welfare. Other philosophers have argued that equal treatment requires equal distribution of certain resources, opportunities, rights and indeed, capabilities. Roughly, all the various propositions for equal treatment can be characterized as falling into one of the three categories of *welfare* (utility, happiness, well-being), *resources* (primary goods, insurance, basic income, opportunities, rights), or *capabilities* (minimum threshold, basic) (Daniels, 1996a).

Despite standing alongside various conceptions or theories of social justice, the reason the CA is referred to as an 'approach' rather than a theory of justice is because it does not have the full components of a general theory of justice. People do indeed disagree about what is necessary for a theory to be considered a complete theory of justice. However, using the work of Rawls as a standard, a theory of justice comprises a political account of the person, a political theory of the good or rights and obligations, a political psychology, and an account of justification that includes the identification of the epistemology and methods used in constructing the theory (Nussbaum, 2006, p. 153).

These components should address the concerns about the coherence of theory construction, the fairness of the proposed conception, and the stability of the theory when being realized in the world. A critique of a theory is often the evaluation of these aspects. Despite having many of these components, the CA is not considered to be a full theory. One reason is that the CA is thought of as not having any 'public criterion of social justice' (Pogge, 2002a, 2010). That is, according to Thomas Pogge, the CA provides a useful language to assess the justness of other theories and real-world situations but, by itself, the CA offers no criterion for what justice should substantively entail. Pogge is essentially asking: if equal treatment is meant to be in the space of capabilities then, capabilities of what? Without any content of capabilities, it is only an analytical framework, not a substantive theory. While it may be possible to answer Pogge's questions, as he seems to completely bypass Nussbaum's arguments for basic capabilities, they still will not transform the CA into a full theory for a number of reasons.

Pursuing an answer to Pogge's question brings us to one of the distinctive aspects of the CA. The CA has two prominent advocates – Amartya Sen and Martha Nussbaum. They developed the approach together for a period of time, but then have gone on to develop it differently. The answer to Pogge's question, and whether the CA is classified as an approach or theory may possibly depend on which of the two versions one pursues. In Sen's case, his initial critique of the focus of welfare economics on utility and Rawls' standardized set of primary goods formed the foundation of the CA. He has recently written that it is neither necessary nor sufficient to have an all-encompassing ideal, 'transcendental' theory in order to evaluate and do justice in particular situations (Sen, 2006, 2009, pp. 96–106).

This seems to imply that his version of the CA does not need to be a comprehensive theory of justice, whatever that may entail, in order to help guide the social realization of justice. Moreover, aside from describing the analytical concept of a capability and how it may be applied to a particular quality of life issue, he has steadfastly refused to identify a 'fixed' list of capabilities that every human being should possess in a conception of a just society. This seems to preclude his version from providing any 'public criterion of justice' that Pogge claims is needed for a theory of justice.

Sen provides a number of reasons for refusing to identify 'the list' of capabilities. One is that the commitment to self-determination and democratic processes in liberal philosophy militates against any specification of the good, or what constitutes the good life. He argues that specifying capabilities would be limiting the contribution of public reasoning and the formation of social values through such a process. Sen also argues that the justification of ethical principles such as the content of capabilities lies in their identification through public deliberation and ability to withstand public scrutiny (Sen, 2009, parts I and II). Nevertheless, Sen himself acknowledges that throughout his writings he has identified what he believes would be some 'basic capabilities' that would be likely to be common across communities when deliberating on the content and priorities of capabilities. These basic capabilities include capabilities for mobility, to live disease-free lives, to satisfy nutritional requirements, to be clothed and sheltered; to participate in the social life of community, and others (Sen, 2004a).

Importantly, Sen argues that a full list of capabilities should not and cannot be identified across human beings because of the plurality and incommensurability of moral goods (Sen, 1994, 2000). Even where democratic processes and public reasoning attempt to identify a list of capabilities, it may be untenable to expect an agreement on a complete and ordered list because of incommensurate values.

In contrast, Nussbaum has pursued constructing a capabilities based theory of justice, which she explicitly identifies as being a 'partial' theory of justice. Nussbaum shares Sen's belief that the 'capability space' is the right place to evaluate the quality of life of individuals and inequalities across individuals. However, she parts with Sen by providing an explicit account of 'core human entitlements' that should be 'respected and implemented by governments of all nations, as a bare minimum of what respect for human dignity requires' (Nussbaum, 2000b, p. 12, 2006, p. 70). Thus, Nussbaum has combined the evaluative space with substantive content, which then is advocated as producing basic political principles for social organization. In following

Rawls' standard of theory construction, she also identifies a necessary moral psychology that consists of greater beneficence and compassion than what is required by dominant social contract theories based on mutual advantage. She also identifies an epistemology and method of using wide reflective equilibrium to move from an intuitive conception of the human being and dignity to the capability entitlements that attach. And she follows Rawls in seeing her theory as being limited to political liberalism, and making the ten central capabilities the object of overlapping consensus in order to provide stability.

What distinguishes Nussbaum's approach from Sen's is that she has identified ten 'central human capabilities' (CHCs), and adds the components of dignity and political liberalism. These capabilities are to be guaranteed by every society to each citizen and, moreover, she writes that 'humanity is under a collective obligations to find ways of living and cooperating together so that all human beings can have decent lives' (Nussbaum, 2006, p. 280). Nussbaum's conception is presented as only a partial theory of justice because she is concerned 'only' with sufficiency, or ensuring minimal thresholds of central capabilities. However, she argues that for some capabilities to be sufficient they will have to be equal. And ensuring sufficient capabilities is seen as one, but not the only, central purpose of social cooperation (Nussbaum, 2006, pp. 71, 75, 274). Because she does not consider establishing all political principles or guiding other social goals, or addressing inequalities in capabilities above the sufficiency thresholds, Nussbaum suggests her partial theory is compatible with other theories of justice being implemented when everyone is above the minimum thresholds levels (Nussbaum, 2000b, p. 12, 2006, p. 75).

One of the drawbacks of the CA is that there is much confusion in the literature about basic concepts, including the idea of a capability. Some of this confusion is due to the differences between Sen and Nussbaum, and some of it is also due to the variety of concepts in different disciplines. Putting aside outright misunderstandings of the idea of capability, choosing to privilege Sen's or Nussbaum's conception over the other, or instead, attempting to bring together both versions as I think one should, requires a thorough understanding of the sources, the distinct forms of both versions, and what they have in common. Even this, however, is not an easy task and is made even more complicated by increasing variations of the capabilities approach.

A few years ago, the simplest distinction between Sen's and Nussbaum's approaches was to consider the Senian version as a descriptive framework while viewing Nussbaum's conception as a normative framework. Sen's approach has been described as providing an analytical device in contrast to Nussbaum's account of substantive entitlements (Alkire, 2005b; Robeyns, 2005a, 2006). This distinction is too weak to hold, however, as Sen's argument also has normative intentions. He argues that for any theory of social justice to be plausible, it has to have some component of treating every person equally in some respect. He further argues that the most defensible conception of equal treatment from the perspective of social justice or equity is to ensure equal or equitable capabilities (Sen, 1992a, 1999a). And lastly, he has clearly stated that though capabilities by themselves do not constitute justice, they are a central part of assessing justice (Sen, 2010). Thus, like Nussbaum, Sen also intends his 'approach' or version of the CA to stand alongside other liberal theories of justice.

Sen's analytical device, quadrants, vectors

The concepts of a capability and functionings have been described in a variety of ways (Sen, 1983; Nussbaum, 2000b; Alkire, 2005b; Robeyns, 2005a, 2006; Vizard, 2006). And, indeed, I have my own contribution to make towards understanding the concept of capabilities and functionings. The simplest way of describing a capability is to say that it is what a person is able to be and do. But, as someone interested in health, I am particularly interested in the embodiment of capabilities. I would like there to be as little distance as possible between theoretical conceptualizations and entitlements to capabilities and the embodied capabilities of human beings. The current models are too grounded in the discipline of economics. They try to show economists how capabilities relate to commodities, characteristics of commodities, and utility or welfare achieved from using commodities. In aiming to create a capability framework for health professionals and non-economists, I believe it is helpful to identify a number of conceptual dyadic distinctions. One may initially conceptualize the idea of a capability as an equation, imagining an archetype capability on one side and on the other side, the personal features/needs and external, physical and social conditions.

For example, a conception of an ideal capability to be well nourished would be on one side of the equals sign and the personal features of the individual and her external conditions on the other. We would want to see whether the combination of the personal features (needs, endowments, conversion skills) and external conditions (physical, social) could come together to constitute real practical opportunity for the person to achieve adequate nutrition; does it approximate the notion of the capability we have in mind on the other side? A capability of achieving a single functioning, such as being sufficiently nourished, is obviously a simplistic example of capability, and really works only in theory. Any human capability is likely to be made up of a cluster of iterative and interactive functionings and capabilities. For example, my getting up and walking from this chair to the door really is made up of complicated, interactive and iterative internal processes, starting at the sub-molecular level and going up to combining with the conditions of my immediate external environment. My capability of walking to the door is an assessment of an entire cluster of complicated capabilities and functionings.

A second dyadic distinction the CA literature frequently discusses is that between capability and functioning. A capability, as previously described, is the practical possibility of exercising or achieving a functioning. The necessity of making such a distinction is grounded in the central value of having opportunity; being able to choose how to pursue one's life. The third dyadic distinction is between the individual's personal features and external physical and social conditions. Some of the CA literature simplifies this distinction as being internal, versus external aspects of capability. But for practical purposes, and to clearly identify where and to what extent social intervention can occur, it may be much more helpful to distinguish clearly the four components: personal features/needs, conversion skills, external physical conditions and social conditions.

The fourth dyadic distinction is between well-being and agency functionings. Nussbaum does not make this distinction, but Sen and those who follow him do. All acts carried out by a person are not necessarily beneficial to the person. Sabina Alkire presents the example of a person A enjoying a picnic who jumps into a frigid river to save another person B in distress (Alkire, 2005b). Jumping into the cold river was not immediately beneficial to person A enjoying the picnic, but she nevertheless, was able to carry out the act. The act of jumping in the river to help B illustrates A's agency functioning but it would not evidence A's well-being functioning. So there is an important distinction to be made between acts that are 'beneficial to' or 'good for' the person acting, and acts that are done for 'other purposes'. In the CA, acts beneficial to the actor are referred to as 'well-being functionings'. They include mental and physical states of the person which are both subjectively and objectively positively valued. And acts aimed for other purposes are referred to as 'agency functionings'.

Agency functionings are intended to encompass the full breadth of acts that individuals undertake in determining, revising and pursuing their conception of the good life. There is seen to be value in being able to have capabilities of exercising both types of functionings. However, the literature suggests that agency functionings make up a much larger category than well-being functionings, and that agency functionings are crucial to realizing well-being functionings.[21] The importance of making this distinction and of showing their inter-dependence relates to debates about the priority of welfare rights versus civil and political liberties. Agency rights are seen to be crucial to securing well-being (Sen, 1981c, 1985b).

All of these various dyadic relationships come together in Sen's version of the CA, where a capability is conceived as having four dimensions or vectors. They include (a) agency-freedom; (b) agency-achievement; (c) well-being freedom; (d) well-being achievement (Sen, 1999a; Alkire, 2005b). For any meaningful capability, these four dimensions identify the importance of there being ability or 'effective freedom' in terms of breadth of extant opportunities and abilities to choose to follow any of them. Importantly, this four-quadrant, multi-dimensionality of any given capability is said to exhibit 'internal plu-rality' for assessing capabilities. Equal capabilities do not mean identical vectors but that there are equal 'effective freedoms' to achieve the functionings across individuals.

As I stated earlier, Nussbaum does not identify a distinction between well-being and agency, but does make use of the distinction between freedoms and achievements, or capabilities and functionings. Her rea-soning for not using such a distinction is based on the potential for confusion caused by the term 'well-being', which has historically been closely associated with utilitarianism. She sees no additional benefits in highlighting or separating well-being from agency functionings that could not be handled within the distinction between capabilities and functionings (Nussbaum, 2000b, p. 14). In fact, Nussbaum categorizes capabilities as being basic, internal, or combined (Nussbaum, 2000b, pp. 84–85). Basic capabilities refer to those biological and mental processes that occur without conscious choice as part of a biological viability. Combined capabilities are those which entail internal capa-bilities combining with suitable external material goods and social conditions in order to exercise a function.

The difference between Nussbaum and Sen on the importance of agency and well-being distinction lies, perhaps, in their different primary disciplines. Sen is supremely concerned with how to make comparisons among individuals about their quality of life. The impossibility of making interpersonal comparisons of utility has been a long-standing problem in neo-classical economics. What Sen has achieved, and is committed to asserting, is that though one might not be able to make interpersonal utility comparisons, we can make comparisons of people in each of the four quadrants. Adherents to the Senian conception of capabilities are asked to think of each capability as being multi-dimensional and more practically, to conceive of each quadrant as a vector contributing to the capability. This allows for understanding that different vectors or quadrants may be able to compensate for the weakness of one or more of the other vector/quadrants in order to reach the achievement. In contrast, Nussbaum's primary grounding in ancient and modern philosophy motivates her reasoning for a conception of human flourishing and its relation to social justice. She does not go into detail about measurement and evaluation of capabilities.

A fifth and final dyadic distinction needs to be identified. Within agency functionings, or acts that are not directly or immediately beneficial to the individual, Sen makes a further distinction between what he calls 'control' and 'effective power' (Sen, 1985b, pp. 208–213). This serves to distinguish between a person's interest in controlling the process that aims to achieve a goal versus the emphasis on achieving the goal even if or when the person does not have direct control over the process. In either situation the person has the capability of achieving the goal, but the person's interest can either be on the *acting* or mechanisms in the first, or the *achieving* in the second. For a myriad of simple and complex functionings, a person may not be able to have control over the process of exercising a functioning, or making it possible to exercise a functioning. Philip Pettit refers to this second kind of functioning achievements as 'indirect liberty' and 'passive empowerment' (Pettit, 2001).

Consider the situation where a child is bathed, a disabled person is carried up the steps, or new laws to restrict air pollution allow one to breathe easier. In each of these examples, the individual achieves functionings, though they could not control the mechanisms or process to the achievement. At a prior point in time, however, they each possessed a capability of achieving the functioning. Referring back to the four vectors, a person not having agency-freedom over the process may be viewed as being less important than the achieving of the well-being functioning. In regard to some functionings, however, it may be much more important that the individual have the well-being freedom. For example, performing surgery on a person to remove a cancerous growth may produce a well-being achievement, but their freedom to choose to have that operation may have significant ethical weight.

In his most recent writings Sen appears to have transformed his concern with the effect of power into 'opportunity freedom' and control into 'process freedom' (Sen, 2009, pp. 228–230). He then links the distinction between the two to the difference between pursuing a culmination outcome, meaning the achievement, versus a comprehensive outcome which aims to take into account the process and achievement (Sen, 2009, pp. 215–217, 228–230). This distinction between culmination and comprehensive outcomes takes on greater significance in Sen's recent writings as he seeks to reclaim consequentialism from the utilitiarians. While eschewing utility or welfare for being culmination outcomes as well as maximization, he argues that CA advocates can and should be consequentialists through aiming to realize comprehensive outcomes. To summarize, it has been suggested that CA becomes easier to understand from five dyadic conceptual distinctions.

1. ideal capability vs. personal features and external conditions
2. capability vs. functionings
3. personal features vs. external physical and social conditions
4. well-being vs. agency functionings
5. control vs. effective power

Nussbaum's CHCs

Nussbaum's initial interest in the CA is motivated by the observations of ancient philosophers such as Aristotle that the focus of moral concern should not be on commodities but on what individuals are able to be and do (Nussbaum, 1987). She saw the same observations in the research and arguments of Sen about capabilities. Sen and Nussbaum originally overlapped in their approaches and shared the theoretical critique of Rawlsian primary goods and utilitarianism (Nussbaum and Sen, 1993). Since then, they have developed separate accounts, and the most significant difference between the two is her explicit account of certain central human capabilities as being pre-political entitlements (Nussbaum, 2000b pp. 11–15). Thus, Pogge's assertion that the CA has no public criteria of justice is directly contradicted by Nussbaum's list of capabilities. As outlined in Chapter 1, Nussbaum maintains that all societies should ensure that every member achieves a certain threshold of some central capabilities. The ten CHCs are seen to be pre-political entitlements which then identify some basic political principles for organizing a minimally just, liberal society (Nussbaum 2006, p. 70).

Nussbaum clearly identifies that the social goal is normally to ensure that individuals have capabilities and not to induce their achievements ('functionings') unless dignity is at stake. And, for children, the social goal should be the achievement of functionings. Capabilities, not functionings are the focus for adults because of the necessity to respect the choices of citizens to determine their own lives, and importantly for Nussbaum, in order to achieve global overlapping consensus on her list of ten CHCs.

Nussbaum's list of CHCs is significantly influenced by Aristotle and Marx, and is centred on the concept of moral worth and human dignity. That is, she conceives of a human being's dignity as being uniquely constituted by its animality, neediness, sociability and ability to reason. Unlike dignity based on moral or prudential reasoning powers of human beings, Nussbaum sees dignity in the human animal which is needy, sociable and capable of reason. She starts from the intuitive idea that certain basic functionings are so central to human life that their absence or presence reflects the absence or presence of human life form. From there, the Marxian component is reflected in recognizing that to be 'fully human' requires that the person does these functionings differently from what would be normal for other animals.

Bringing together Aristotle, Marx and some aspects of Grotius, Nussbaum argues that a life worthy of the dignity of the human being is made up of opportunity and activity that reflects the neediness, sociability and ability to reason of the human animal. That is, these functions are not done purely by animal instincts or through being passively shaped and pushed around by nature and accident, but infused throughout by reasoning, cooperation and reciprocity with other human beings (Nussbaum, 2000b, p. 72).

Her list of basic capabilities, contrary to some cursory criticisms, does not advocate a form of an ideal human being or 'perfectionism' (Arneson, 2000; Nussbaum, 2000a). Unlike others who do advocate a version of Aristotelian perfectionism, Nussbaum argues for minimum threshold levels of central capabilities. These levels of capability or opportunity ensure that each human being is able to pursue diverse conceptions of life, in a way worthy of the dignity of the human being. The list of ten CHCs does not describe a comprehensive conception of the good life for every human being. Rather, the list of basic capabilities identifies a minimal level of freedom, thresholds of capabilities and functionings, which every society should ensure to its citizens. Beneath these thresholds, human beings do not have basic functionings which allow for a life worthy of the dignity of being human.

A second criticism that has been directed at the list of ten CHCs and the CA in general is that it constrains possible conceptions of the good (Nussbaum, 1999, part I). The list is said to be patently illiberal for specifying and valuing certain content of a life. Nussbaum has been open in taking a position that a commitment to liberalism does indeed involve making some minimal normative commitments to a conception of the good. The charge that the CA or CHCs constrain the conception of the good for human beings also depends on how critics believe human agents come to have the rationality to conceive their life plans and where ethical theory should begin. For example, Rawls avoids this problem largely by requiring from the start that his hypothetical contractors have full rationality. That is, his 'thin theory of the good' requires that individuals be rational in order to conceive their life plans, and have a sense of justice. Their capacity for impartiality is reflected in the use of the veil of ignorance.

Moreover, in order for there to be any interest in making a contract, individuals must be free, equal, independent, and in an environment of moderate scarcity. For Rawls, the representatives behind the veil of ignorance embody the minimum conception of the person, and what they seek to achieve. Having such a scenario of contractors in mind, a list of central human capabilities may seem to be superimposing on the rational capacities of individuals to determine their own lives. However, if we compare what Rawls requires of his moral agents in terms of each being free, equal, independent, having two moral powers, and with impartiality provided by the veil with the minimum level of opportunity and activity Nussbaum seeks to ensure through the ten CHCs, there is not such a big difference in either of their 'thin' theories of the good. Nussbaum does not identify any more capabilities than those Rawls requires for his contract procedure to get off the ground.

Nussbaum could reply to the charge of ethical imperialism by stating that the list is neither a final nor a complete account, but a minimal account of activity and opportunity in a human life. If, however, critics believe that the list of ten CHCs could force individuals to be and do what they would not choose if they were fully free and independent, rational agents, the charge may have some impact. Nussbaum's commitment to liberal principles leads her to argue that the list of ten CHCs does require making negative judgements on certain practices and beliefs that violate the equal respect and concern for individuals. The ten CHCs, at the least, allow people to have a real choice in deciding whether to limit some of their own capabilities, and preserve an exit option from situations where their capabilities are limited (Nussbaum, 2000b, pp. 91–96).[22] Some functionings may be so valuable to maintaining minimal human dignity that they will not be allowed to be neglected or fail, even if it means overriding individual choice. Moreover, certain functionings–achievements may require collective provision, or public goods, thus it is forthrightly admitted that there will be some areas where individuals do not have control over the exact mechanisms or processes of achieving functionings.

Aside from the prevalent criticisms that the capability list is perfectionist or that it constrains conceptions of the good, a secondary line of criticism has been that the list does not prioritize among the ten capabilities. Going against the received view that any list of moral goods that are to be provided as a matter of justice have to be ranked or indexed into a single metric, Nussbaum vehemently asserts that the ten capabilities are not open to trade-offs (Nussbaum, 2006, pp. 166–167). Every single one of the ten capabilities is an important aspect of a dignified human being, and the foremost social goal is to ensure every citizen is above the threshold for each. She is clear, however, that the entitlements provide political principles only up to the point where all citizens achieve various thresholds of basic human capabilities. Perhaps, ranking or weighting of capabilities will be required or compatible with a theory of justice above the thresholds. Where not all capabilities can be supported, perhaps in the short term, it should simply be recognized that justice is not yet being done on the path towards ensuring sufficient capabilities.

Nussbaum's ten CHCs, as they partly provide a source for political principles for a pluralistic liberal society, are meant to serve as the basis of national constitutions (Nussbaum, 2006, pp. 69–81). And, aside from providing the political principles for domestic governments, the list of basic human capabilities is aimed also to provide coherence and philosophical justification for a basic set of international human rights. Nussbaum has argued that because the CHCs are derived from a conception of a life worthy of the dignity of a human being, it is a species-wide conception. Duties and obligations in regard to supporting basic capabilities of non-compatriots would be more expansive than today and what is being advocated by modern social contract theorists, but still less than what would be required within national borders (Nussbaum, 2006).

Criticisms of the CA

Someone either misunderstanding the CA or mounting an objection could say that a profound flaw in the CA is that it considers someone to have a capability whether or not they have control over the process of realizing the capability. In essence, such an attack directed at the Senian CA would be that if a capability is indeed understood as the total combination of four vectors, then the 'achievement' vectors could compensate for the freedom vectors. Thus, 'achievements' which can really just be social inducements of certain well-being or agency functionings would still be considered as the person having capabilities. Another objection could be that even if the CA asserts stringent criteria for determining which functionings can be induced, just the privileging of certain capabilities over others is still dangerous. Social arrangements can go a long way towards encouraging or endorsing certain kinds of beings and doings without actually forcing or inducing an individual directly to be and do certain things. It is the government inducement of capabilities or 'capacities' and 'equality of capacities' that Dworkin finds frightening (Dworkin, 2000 , p. 302).

Against this criticism of the Senian capability device, one may also be able better to appreciate the almost automatic challenge to Nussbaum's ten CHCs as being oppressive, or illiberal. Surely, given incommensurable conceptions of the good, conflicts in values, and necessity for respecting diversity in the contemporary world, identifying ten things that every human being must be able to be and do is patently illiberal? Against such a broad-brushed criticism, Nussbaum mounts a strong defence of her list of ten CHCs. Her conception of a person which she has in mind with those ten capabilities is not very different from the implicit conceptions in competing theories including in Rawls' theory, and perhaps, even in Dworkin's theory (Dworkin, 1993, 2000). Moreover, paternalism and coercion are both unavoidable in organizing large and complex societies, and come to the forefront almost immediately when considering health concerns (O'Neill, 2002c, 2002a, 2002b; Nuffield Council on Bioethics, 2007; Thaler and Sunstein, 2008).

Furthermore, objective assessments and public deliberation on the content of capabilities, including which of them will require the inducement of functionings, the identification of levels and so forth are meant to be constrained by the over-arching respect for dignity and moral worth of human beings. Inducing people into being and doing certain things that undermine their dignity and calling them achievements would be unacceptable within the CA. Engendering choice and opportunity to reason in all aspects of life plans is central to the notion of human capabilities in the CA and Nussbaum's CHCs. Of course, the possibility of abusing the language and ideas of the CA surely exists. Just as rights language can become just a shell for asserting interests, the language of CA also has the potential to be abused. Such potential for abuse should not be seen as an inherent or fatal flaw.

A second objection to the CA comes from exactly the opposite direction. G. A. Cohen argues that Sen and the CA privilege the 'freedom to achieve' more than the actual achievements (Cohen, 1989). Do we care about individuals having freedom to achieve more or equally as much as the individual achieving the functioning; even some basic functionings? Cohen argues that emphasis on freedom more than achievements makes the CA too 'athletic', and proceeds to develop his own theory of entitlements to 'mid-fare'. Mid-fare includes some objective functioning achievements advantageous to human beings as they pursue their own ends. Cohen's critique has been addressed by Philip Pettit, who points to the CA's recognition of what he calls 'passive empowerment' or inducement of functionings, whereby it is not always or only focused on potential achievements (Pettit, 2001).

Nevertheless, there is still a meaningful question regarding the space between a person's possessing the capability and actually achieving the functionings; individuals may have capabilities but not choose to achieve the functionings. Nussbaum is much more forthright in identifying the persuasive role of moral education, restrictions on letting functionings wither, and direct inducements which close this space between availability and achievement. But given that the CA is centrally motivated by human deprivation, and such pressing concerns as the deaths of millions of individuals due to health threats such as HIV/AIDS and other preventable causes, does the CA sufficiently balance our value of both the freedom to achieve and the achievement? That is to say, do we want to give individuals mere opportunity or actually have them be protected? For example, Madison Powers and Ruth Faden develop a theory informed by Sen and Nussbaum but give priority to functionings over capabilities (Powers and Faden, 2008, pp. 37–41). They argue that a principle defining the limits of what others can to do to bring about well-being in individuals does the work better than asserting the priority of capabilities over achievements.

While I think Powers and Faden undervalue opportunity and the respect for choice, they do rightly highlight the breech between capability and functionings. Though the CA has achieved success in expanding the focus of economic and justice theories to include human capabilities, the CA's advocates have not yet begun fully to consider the theoretical and practical issues in the self-realization of capabilities and the process of choosing to exercise capabilities and functionings. What can the CA say about the responsibility or duty to engender one's own capabilities or achieve functionings?

Frontier issues

There are a number of issues that the CA faces which relate to its development rather than criticisms or objections. Thomas Pogge picks up on the foremost question for the CA namely, which capabilities? On the one hand, Sen has repeatedly talked about certain capabilities as being basic, or even asserted the priority of liberty. He has recently tried to ground human rights in the capabilities framework, showing his interest in asserting capabilities as universal entitlements (Sen, 2004c).

Richard Arneson puts further pressure on Sen by using Sen's criticisms of welfarism against him. Arneson, picking up on the CA's critique of using preferences to measure advantage or well-being then argues that without an objective account of capabilities, letting individuals choose their own capabilities is the same as a theory which relies on preferences (Arneson, 2010). He argues that there has to be an objective list of capabilities. In comparison, Nussbaum strongly asserts that the list of ten CHCs should be ensured in their entirety, and are applicable to all members of the human species.

However, Nussbaum's process of justification or achieving overlapping consensus on the list is not delimited in any way. The open-ended process, occurring at a global level, striving to achieve global overlapping consensus, seems to make the justification only tentative, if it could be fully achieved ever at all. Given that reflective equilibrium is not just an affirmation process, but a truly dialectical process, there is no assurance that the list we have now is the one that will achieve through overlapping consensus. So, how will Sen, Nussbaum and others committed to the CA proceed in identifying the content of capabilities?

A point related to the content of capabilities is the question of measurement and weights. Sen identifies multiple dimensions or vectors for each capability, but there is still a lot of theoretical and empirical work to be done on developing methods to measure these dimensions. It cannot be overstated how important measurements are given that what we measure has to reflect exactly the importance CA gives to distinguishing between effective freedom and functioning-achievement as well as well-being and agency. Some progress has been made on identifying the multi-dimensionality of capabilities and development of a variety of measurement tools (Chiappero-Martinetti and Roche, 2009).

Nussbaum, on the other hand, avoids the four vectors approach and distinguishes only between capabilities and functionings (Nussbaum,

2000b, p. 14). She believes that such a distinction is sufficient to handle the various aspects of effective freedom the CA is concerned about. However, such a version may be even more difficult to measure given the greater room for interpretation. Nevertheless, even Nussbaum's list has been taken up by empirical researchers, particularly in the domain of health (Anand et al., 2005; Coast et al., 2008a).

A second measurement question pertains to the weights given to different capabilities. That is, how does one rank different capabilities not only in terms of lexical priority, but with different weighting to better capture how much more or less important a capability is than the one below or above it? For Nussbaum, this problem is simple, as she rejects the separation or selecting out certain capabilities from the ten CHCs. All the CHCs must be provided to every human being. However, asserting that all ten CHCs must be present does not mean each has to be present in the same amount or weight. The capability for play must be present, but does it have to be present in the same 'amount' as the capability for bodily integrity? But even more problematic is that the ten CHCs are not singular, unidirectional functioning.

Every embodied functioning is a complicated, iterative set of functionings and capabilities that can keep being peeled away all the way down to the processes at the sub-molecular level. So the question of measurements and weights is a concern not only at the level of ten capabilities but also within each capability. Interestingly, though Sen's arguments for capabilities does not directly go to the weights issue because he does not identify any particular capabilities as valuable, he has, nevertheless, expounded on the difficulties of measurements, particularly in reference to health capability (Sen, 1998a, 2001b, 2002a).

Considering content, measures and weights of capabilities goes directly to concerns about implementation. While it is true that the CA has been the basis for measuring quality of life such as in the United Nations Human Development Reports, aside from references to the theory, the actual use of the concepts has been fairly minimal. Moreover, the articulated aim of the CA and ten CHCs as possible bases for international human rights law and national constitutions is ambitious. But how one gets there is unclear. The hurdles range from the complexity of the theory, and the lack of overlapping consensus, to the issues in realizing political theory, more generally. And perhaps, even more foundational to implementation is the question of whether the CA is an approach to evaluating quality of life; is it a partial theory of justice, or is it still developing into a full theory of justice? Indeed, for Nussbaum, the ten CHCs are a moral minimum, making it a partial theory of justice. Nevertheless, she argues, achieving the moral minimum for every human being is such an overwhelming task that it is not a weakness to defer identifying whether equality of full capabilities or some other social goals come next.

Conclusion

Needless to say, this discussion has only been a cursory introduction to the CA. There are numerous books and academic articles on the approach. Rather than recapitulate the history and content of the CA, the main purpose of this chapter was to provide the background for the next chapter, where the CH argument is presented. It is a hybrid argument as it brings together the analytical structure of Sen's CA and famine entitlement-analysis with Nussbaum's CHCs. Sen's refusal to identify any basic capabilities across human beings precludes using his conception of capabilities for a species-wide conception of human health. No capability, or a minimal account of a life and the good, is concretely identified as being shared across every member of the human species.

In contrast, Nussbaum's fully evaluative conception of human life form and its grounding in human dignity provides justifiable entitlements for every member of the human species (Nussbaum, 2006, pp. 181–183). But Nussbaum does not ground her central capabilities in any causal theory. Chapters 1 and 2 were aimed to show how Nussbaum's ethical argument fits in with the existing debates on the philosophy of health, as well as explicate a theory of causation and distribution of health capability that is more coherent than existing theories in epidemiology. The next chapter discusses the CH argument and shows how it brings together Sen's analysis of the causality of capability sets and the capability device itself with Nussbaum's content and justification for central human capabilities and functionings.

4

The Capability to
be Healthy

The capability to be healthy (CH) is a person's ability to achieve or exercise a cluster of basic capabilities and functionings, and each at a level that constitutes a life worthy of equal human dignity in the modern world. Making use of Nussbaum's theory of central human capabilities (CHCs), the CH can be usefully understood as a 'meta-capability' to achieve or exercise ten CHCs. These ten CHCs together make up a minimal conception of a fully human life, and provide the bases for determining the decent social minimum of entitlements in the relevant parts of an individual's life (Nussbaum, 2000b, p. 75). I also follow Nussbaum's reasoning that these ten basic capabilities of human beings 'are sources of moral claims *wherever* (italics mine) we find them: they exert a moral claim that they should be developed and given a life that is flourishing rather than stunted' (Nussbaum, 2006, p. 278). As a result of seeing health as a capability and relying on Nussbaum's theory for the content of the capability, the CH is a human species-wide ethical conception of health, as well as a source of moral claims for human beings wherever human beings are found; it is a conception of a human right to the capability to be healthy.

The cluster of ten basic, inter-dependent and iterative capabilities and functionings reflect the biology and physiology of the human organism as well as including other capabilities and functionings which reflect the neediness, sociability and capacity for reasoning of the human animal. It is not a theory based on what human nature is or what entitlements arise from that nature. Nor is it a natural-law theory expounding self-evident truths about human needs. Rather, the cluster of capabilities describes a fully evaluative and ethical conception of the human being. Scientific knowledge about the human being provides information about what a human being is, what she can do, what vulnerabilities and limitations she can experience, her life cycle, and so forth. Such empirical knowledge about the nature of the human being alone does not tell us what to value about the human being. For that, we rely on free-standing ethical reasoning about dignity, freedom and equality of human beings in the modern world.

A person who has all the ten CHCs, each above a certain threshold level, has a life of activity and opportunity that represents a life that is fully human. As such, it is clearly not a conception of a life that is just barely human, or even that of an ideal human life. A fully human life is a notion of a human life possessing a sufficient level of opportunity and activity for achieving reasonable and diverse conceptions of the good life (Nussbaum, 2006, p. 182). What should also be emphasized is that a conception of a capability to be healthy as being constituted by a life with a sufficient level of opportunity and choice does not deny the moral worth of lives with less than sufficient capabilities; it does not say that such lives are not worth living, or that they are not human. Such a conception also does not say that there does not exist any freedom, opportunity or agency beneath the sufficient thresholds. Indeed, millions of human beings are attempting to live their lives with insufficient capabilities. Instead, the moral entitlement to a CH is an ethical argument that individuals with insufficient capabilities are being denied their equal human dignity; they are not being given or treated with equal respect which is reflected in their lack of sufficient capabilities.

The CH as well as any human capability is reflected in the interaction of a person's unique biological endowments and needs, external physical and social conditions and agency. Such a notion of agency includes 'conversion skills' that can help convert endowments and external conditions into functionings. Material conditions such as availability of healthcare and adequate nutrition are determined by social arrangements, so material goods come under social conditions. And, if we think about a theory of social justice as informing us what to distribute and how – as providing a metric and distribution rule – then in this case, the metric is the social bases of the capability to be healthy, and the rule is up to the level that is commensurate with equal human dignity in the modern world. Claims for social support for the CH work through the social bases of each of the causal, constitutive components of the CH – endowments and needs, external physical and social conditions and conversion skills.

Furthermore, a moral claim to social support to achieve a sufficient level of CH is not only a claim to material resources but also entails other kinds of claims involving powers, privileges and immunities. For example, the ability to achieve various functionings, such as avoiding a fatal infection, may require a material good like a vaccine. However, where such a vaccine does not exist, having control over one's body and behaviour, and the immediate physical environment in order to prevent infection entails various kinds of powers, privileges, and immunities. The close link between the idea of sufficiency and equal human dignity means that not only is the distribution of CH a concern, but also the causes, persistence, consequences of ill-health and possibilities for social action. Two individuals with the same but less than sufficient levels of CH may have different kinds of moral claims because of different dimensions of each individual's CH. Furthermore, the variety of claims arising from each capability can also be directed at different agents, involve different duties with different levels of obligation.

Ethical and political justification

The argument for the CH presented in this book is an extension of the CA, and indeed, is a hybrid argument that draws on both Sen's and Nussbaum's reasoning. Because it extends the CA, I do not attempt to offer full justification for the CA but rely and build on what has already been done previously. Indeed, there are quite interesting and difficult issues regarding how one justifies ethical theories, compares different theories, or how deep one has to dig into fundamental concepts before starting to build an argument about social justice. For a meaningful justification of the CA one must look first-hand at the most recent writings of Sen and Nussbaum (Nussbaum, 2000b, 2006; Sen, 2009, 2010). What needs justifying in the CA at the level of meta-ethics is the fundamental value that is given to freedom or capability and, in Nussbaum's case, the entitlements to ten CHCs. Asserting freedom, dignity and capability as having or being of fundamental value in a theory then allows the building up of the analysis that can constantly refer back to how freedom or dignity is being affected.

So, one can reason that a move will be good or bad for freedom, or one theory is good or bad for dignity, and so forth. If one disagrees with freedom or dignity as being a fundamental value then it is hard to go along with the analysis. Sen, Nussbaum and others provide various kinds of arguments, some analytical and some ethical, and they identify methodologies of reasoning which provide justification and stability to such starting points and the consequent analysis. The disagreement over fundamental values is why this book presented arguments in Part I that supported the idea of health as capability, and the science of the social bases of health capability. They provide support outside of the CA, to show those who might not agree with the fundamental value of capability, that the CA is supported by philosophy of health arguments and epidemiological science. They show the stability of the argument for the CH and the CA.

This is not the place to discuss extensively the justification of the CA. But briefly, in order to be transparent about my own position, I must note that I presently rely heavily on Nussbaum's justification of the account of central human capabilities. I find her method of 'political justification' to be more immediately plausible than the highly demanding and yet open-textured process of justification that Sen advocates involving public reasoning, participatory social decision-making, rationality, impartiality, and objectivity (Sen, 2009). By no means am I saying that these are not important and relevant ideas. Rather, they are ideas that still require closer consideration. In contrast, Nussbaum's account of political justification is more immediately accessible as it is based on that of John Rawls, which is in turn informed by that of Charles Larmore (Larmore, 1987; Rawls, 1993; Larmore, 1996; Nussbaum, 2001).

In Nussbaum's account, like that of Rawls, the method of justification is a process of reasoning that confronts one's own considered moral judgements with a range of relevant theoretical views and principles. Through a dialectical process of reasoning the aim is to find a stable fit between one's considered judgements and principles and theories through adjusting either side appropriately. And this process is not done alone but 'Socratically', among members of a political community, and about the reasonable terms of social cooperation. The burden lies on the interlocutor to show that what is being put forward could, over time, be the basis of an overlapping consensus among members. That is, we do not have to show that it definitely will attain such overlapping consensus but, rather, identify a plausible path towards achieving that overlapping consensus. This is, at least, how I understand Nussbaum's account of political justification.

The great advantage of simply extending an established theory or approach to social justice is that one can stand on the shoulders of giants; most of the difficult work at justification is already done. In trying to put health into the centre of social justice, I have so far been aiming to follow a similar methodology to that of Nussbaum by showing how health can be coherently conceived as a capability, outlining how it is created and distributed, arguing for how such a capability gives rise to moral claims and lastly, confronting this conception with alternative approaches to health claims particularly those focusing on welfare and resources. In fact, aside from alternative ethical approaches, I have also confronted the ethical ideas with scientific theories and principles. I contrasted my conception of health with the dominant scientific conception, showed why it is more coherent, and have proposed a theory of causation and distribution of capabilities as being a more coherent explanatory paradigm for epidemiology.

The fit between the arguments for CH and empirical, scientific principles and theories should provide more 'stability' in addition to the ethical reasoning about moral claims to CHCs. All of these components build a plausible pathway, over time, towards achieving overlapping consensus on a conception of a moral right to the CH; an overlapping consensus on conceiving human health as an assessment of a person's capability of exercising at least ten basic capabilities and functionings, and that this conception of health is a source of moral claims for social support and protection for human beings wherever we find them.

CH as pre-political moral entitlement

Nussbaum's ten CHCs are grounded in a freestanding conception of human dignity. Therefore, because the CH is seen as meta-capability to achieve these ten CHCs, so too is the present conception of the CH grounded in dignity. The argument is that every human being has claims to social support arising from the dignity of the human being as an inherently 'needy temporal animal being' (Nussbaum, 2006, p. 160). For Nussbaum, there is further importance in recognizing the difference between capabilities as instrumental to achieving a life with dignity versus capabilities creating dignity within 'areas of life human beings typically engage' (Nussbaum, 2006, p. 161). By pointing to such a subtle difference she wants to establish a theory of the good prior to any social agreement or political principles. An instrumental notion of capabilities would make her theory similar to contract theories that build structures to distribute valued goods. By interweaving a conception of human dignity and central human capabilities without one being prior to another, she is able to argue that a life worthy of human dignity gives rise to pre-political moral entitlements to the central human capabilities. Because capabilities and dignity are mutually constitutive, the list of CHCs is a freestanding theory of the good (Nussbaum, 2006, pp. 160–164).

Such an account of the CHCs is thus enormously helpful for an argument for the CH because it also allows for a species-wide conception of human health. Every member of the human species is covered under such a conception, and it identifies the bases of a moral entitlement prior to any social contract or other types of political agreements. Such pre-political entitlements therefore, impact the theoretical landscape of global justice which I discuss in Chapter 7. Furthermore, health or the CH is not valued primarily because of its instrumental value, but first and foremost, because of its intrinsic value as constituting human dignity and well-being.

Health and CA

The argument for the CH is partly motivated by the need to address the CA's currently ambiguous conception of health capability. Both Sen and Nussbaum have indeed discussed and referred to human health concerns in terms of capabilities. Sen has suggested such a capability in different writings and through his use of various examples of health functionings. And Nussbaum has explicitly identified capabilities related to longevity and 'bodily health' in her argument that every society should guarantee its citizens and residents the social bases to ten central human capabilities. However, the writings of both create much uncertainty about the content of a CH in either of their versions and in the CA more generally. Such an assertion necessarily requires some elucidation. So I start with an illustrative example from Sen. In the seminal monograph *Inequality Re-Examined*, Sen contrasts the subjective welfarist conception of well-being with the 'well-ness' of a person understood as the achievement of a set of interrelated functionings that can include 'being adequately nourished, being in good health, avoiding escapable morbidity and premature mortality, etc. . . .' (1992a, p. 39).

Looking beyond his specific concern to distinguish between subjective well-being and well-ness, his listing of being healthy as a separate functioning from being adequately nourished and avoiding morbidity and premature mortality is confusing. What does he think being in good health is if not avoiding disease and premature mortality? Does he mean being in good vigour aside from avoiding disease? Though this could seen as a one-off instance of ambiguity, Sen's vehement refusal to identify any 'core' or 'basic' capabilities has meant that he has not offered a systematic evaluation or definitive account of any single capability. What we have is his use of examples to buttress the general arguments for the CA in various areas of social concern. I should not be misunderstood as saying that Sen's unwillingness to specify the form and content of *the* capability to be healthy means that he has not extensively discussed health or health capability. It would be grossly mistaken to minimize the extensive consideration Sen has given to preventable mortality and illness and health inequalities.

As the quote in the introductory paragraph to this book evinces, Sen asserts that health is central to social justice, and has been writing extensively on aspects of health, health policy, health inequality and so forth for decades. In fact, in his Tanner Lectures on Human Values titled, *'Equality of What'* given in 1979 and seen as the starting point of the CA, Sen uses the example of a physically disabled individual to critique primary goods and utilitarianism before championing the idea of capabilities (Sen, 1982b). Health or the absence of health has been a major concern, motivating concept, and space to evaluate justice from the beginning. In any case, despite the long-standing concern for health and longevity, there is no comprehensive or definitive Senian argument for what health is, why it is valuable, what entitlements and obligations are related to it, how to address conflicts in entitlements, or how to reason about hard choices. There are general and often insightful explorations, discussions and perhaps what can be seen as useful guidance on different aspects of addressing avoidable ill-health, disability and mortality as well as advancing health equity (Sen, 1981a, 1982b, 1984, 1985a, 1992b, 1992a, 1994, 1998a, 1999c, 1999d, 1999b, 2001b, 2002a, 2002c, 2004a, 2004b, 2006, 2007, 2009).

In contrast, Nussbaum provides a more definitive account of a capability to be healthy in *Women and Human Development* (WHD), (Nussbaum 2000b, pp. 70–96). However, she too leaves a lot undone. In WHD, as part of arguing how certain capabilities are constitutive of human dignity, in specific regard to health capability, Nussbaum points out that there will be a need to determine which health functionings should be induced for various individuals or situations rather than just ensuring the capability as well as the need for determining what threshold levels of all the various functionings must be achieved in order to be considered adequate. For example, she suggests that some capabilities will have to be relatively equal while others have to be above an absolute threshold to be considered sufficient.

Nevertheless, while providing some general outlines, she defers all further discussion about inducing functionings and the minimum threshold levels of functionings to a future legislative stage and public deliberation (Nussbaum, 2000b, p. 91). This deferral is too premature. There are many aspects of the causes, persistence, levels, distribution patterns and differential consequences of health capability achievements and failures that need to be considered in the discussions on first principles of social organization.

Capabilities and severe disability

Nussbaum's argument for a partial theory of social justice is commendable partly for making the interests of individuals who are severely physically and mentally impaired part of the discussions on the basic principles of justice. She emphasizes that taking into account the interests of severely impaired individuals at the first stage of ethical reasoning on basic principles of social justice will result in substantive guidance for the basic structures of society. This is in contrast to considering their interests at the legislative stage when only cursory accommodations will result as the most of the important aspects of society are already fixed. That is, when theories erase human disabilities or assume the full health of moral agents, then the interests of disabled individuals get shunted to a later stage after the basic structure is settled. It is necessary to consider their interests from the start as a matter of social justice, because every individual human being, even when severely impaired, should be treated as an equal member of society. Their interests, and of those who provide them with care, must be considered from the beginning, along with those of all the other human beings who are not severely impaired.

As part of the reasoning she provides, Nussbaum links the state of being severely disabled – being in an unequal status with others due to vulnerability, neediness, and dependence – with the periods of being in ill-health that everyone will experience at one time or another. She wants to establish that human functioning is on a continuum, and every human being can expect to change positions on that continuum during their life cycle. While she articulates the injustice in excluding the interests of those individuals on the extreme ends of the continuum, she does not go further and consider more closely the possible injustice in the causes, persistence through generations, levels, the social distribution of severe impairments, the concept of health being used on her list, or the most current research and theories of causation and distribution of impairments and mortality.

Without such consideration, Nussbaum appears to be accepting that severe impairments are caused randomly or by nature. Perhaps without realizing it, she follows Rawls in accepting that there is a natural baseline or distribution of human functionings, and that severely mentally impaired individuals are in the tails, or below the threshold of the normal range. Yet, her initial insight that only cursory accommodations will be made in the legislative stage rather than substantive ones regarding severely impaired individuals is also relevant when we look more closely at the causation and distribution of severe impairments, and more broadly at the multiple dimensions of health and longevity.

Perhaps the reason Nussbaum does not take the next, further step from severe disability to looking at ill-health more broadly is because her primary concern is representing the interests of severely impaired individuals, and with showing how their role in ideal theorizing reveals a flaw, perhaps a fatal flaw, in the social contract tradition. She has not, as far as I am aware, explored the causes and social distribution patterns of severe impairments; she handles disability as a stable, inherent trait of individuals. That is, like Dworkin, the moral concern is for Tiny Tim as a disabled individual, and without any consideration of the causes of his disability, his group membership or other dimensions. Though Nussbaum is right to advocate for the interests of severely impaired individuals, if severe impairments are socially caused, correlated with or persist in certain social groups then there would be something more to consider aside from the consequences of disability on individuals and their caregivers. For instance, Sen makes the point that only a moderate proportion of the six hundred million disabled individuals in the world presently were doomed to be that way at conception or birth (Sen, 2009, p. 259).

Justice regarding severe impairments should be concerned not only with how individuals who are severely impaired and their carers should be treated, but also be concerned with preventing disabilities and possible offensive correlations in the social distribution of disabilities. When we look at the marked social gradient in avoidable impairments, including severe impairments, as well as their wide-ranging social determinants, it becomes clear that there is much more to consider about health at the initial stage of discussions on first principles of social organization.

One major implication of giving more consideration to health capability, which is particularly relevant to Nussbaum's approach, is that in light of the recent social determinants research and global experience with new and resurgent infectious disease epidemics such as HIV/AIDS or MDR-TB, ensuring the social bases even to just a sufficient threshold level of health capability for every citizen will require a stringent and irrevocable commitment to certain basic social arrangements. Once the state-of-the-art knowledge about causation and distribution of human impairments and mortality is taken into account, Nussbaum's theory cannot be thought of as a partial or minimal account of social justice; social epidemiological research shows that ensuring health and longevity capabilities will require the functioning and fixing of many basic social institutions, processes and values as well as require the perpetual monitoring and management of relative social inequalities because of their impact on health and longevity, especially in wealthy countries.

Nussbaum conceives her list as being a source of political principles up to the point when all individuals have certain threshold levels of capabilities. As a result, it is seen as a theory of sufficient capabilities. But the research from social epidemiology shows that in societies and environments where most people are above sufficiency capability thresholds (e.g. Sweden, Norway) broad social arrangements continue to affect longevity, health and health inequalities (Ostlin and Diderichsen, 2001). As discussed in Chapter 2, this research has illuminated a whole range of social determinants – discrete exposures as well as pathways – to ill-health over the entire life cycle starting from the social conditions surrounding the mother while in-utero to social relationships in old age (Marmot and Wilkinson, 1999; Berkman and Kawachi, 2000).

While the availability of healthcare is one social determinant, other and probably more influential determinants include such things as early infant care and stimulation, safe and secure employment, housing conditions, experiences of discrimination, self-respect, community cohesion, income inequality and so forth. These determinants operate at levels ranging from the micro to the macro, such as material deprivations and psychosocial mechanisms to community cultures, national political regimes and global processes. Thus, in order to ensure that individuals live their full lifespans and avoid preventable disease-related impairments, there will be a need *indefinitely* to regulate or prevent certain social inequalities in order to prevent or mitigate resulting inequalities in health capability. That is, some kinds of social inequalities across individuals and groups should not be allowed because they will affect basic capabilities, and such inequalities should not be allowed even after every individual has the minimum level of central capabilities because they could undermine the maintenance of capabilities above the sufficiency thresholds. This leads to discarding the possible notion of a minimal conception of central capabilities as a water-level mark that needs to be reached through provision of minimal material goods and social conditions. Rather, whatever the level of material and social conditions, ensuring a minimum set of CHCs means that certain kinds of social inequalities cannot be allowed, for they will always threaten to undermine minimum thresholds of CHC or CH. This understanding of social determinants of impairments and mortality as being possible permanent threats to human capabilities casts doubt on Nussbaum's openness to other possible schemes of social justice, such as Rawls' theory, after achieving certain threshold levels of every citizen.

A more thorough appreciation of the causation and distribution of the ten CHCs in light of social determinants' research will more than likely mean that some of the stringent requirements for or against certain social conditions under a capabilities threshold regime will have to be permanent features of societies, or part of any theories applicable above the thresholds. The upshot of this is that Nussbaum's theory for ten central human capabilities is not a minimal theory at all; it fixes society to a great extent below and above any minimal thresholds because of the broad social bases of health and longevity.

In this discussion of health in capabilities theory, the argument of Jennifer Prah Ruger is worth giving some attention because she has developed a unique argument on health and capabilities (Ruger, 2010). Starting from first principles, she argues that the value of health to individuals means that social justice requires applying a 'health capability paradigm' to health policy. And she develops what such a health capability paradigm means for how healthcare, public health goods and health research should be provided. One of the most striking aspects of the theory, given Prah Ruger's emphasis on the fundamental ethical value of health capabilities – in contrast to health outcomes or healthcare – is that she takes a strident position against extending the scope of social action to address health concerns beyond the traditional boundaries of healthcare policy. In particular, despite acknowledging social determinants of health research, Prah Ruger makes the sweeping statement that we are far from understanding the precise societal mechanisms that influence health, and it would be unwise and unfeasible to improve health with sweeping non-healthcare policies (Ruger, 2010, pp. 6, 98–103).

This is an unwarranted dismissal of a significant body of research with some clear findings. It is unclear whether she is raising the philosophical problem of causation in epidemiology and social epidemiology, or if she is saying that it is too premature to make conclusions. Moreover, by dismissing the possibilities of social action beyond healthcare, it is also unclear if Prah Ruger is making the ethical claim that the only social basis to health capability is healthcare, even broadly understood. If she is, then, her theory does not recognize or address the extensive range of health injustices caused by social arrangements aside from the functioning of healthcare. If she is not making that claim, then her theory is incomplete as it only deals with healthcare among a wide range of social bases of health. Healthcare is only a minor determinant of health and longevity. The contrast between social policies which focus only on healthcare policy versus all the social bases of health and longevity should be easy to see. Nevertheless, Prah Ruger seems to be pursuing the line that health capability should be pursued only through what is within the scope of healthcare.

The capability of being healthy

The CH and each CHC within are made up of the independent, inter-active and iterative processes involving a person's unique internal features/needs, external physical conditions, social conditions, and behaviours and conversion skills. As described in Chapter 2, this causal model of the CH reformulates the biomedical model of health which recognizes the causal factors of disease as being genetic endow-ment, individual behaviour and exposure to external pathogenic mate-rials. Such a model in actuality identifies the causes of disease or health constraints rather than health, even health thought of a species typical functioning. It identifies when functioning is not typical, rather than identifying the causes of typical functioning. And, even then, it excludes social causes. The present CH model is concerned with health capabili-ties and is also more explicit about the causation of CHCs than Nuss-baum's heuristic classification of capabilities. She identifies capabilities as being basic, internal, or combined (Nussbaum, 2000b,pp. 84–86). Her analysis of capabilities as either being naturally endowed ready to function, or requiring various kinds of external material and social support is too causally simplistic. Such a descriptive model also creates too firm a distinction between personal features and external material and social conditions.

When examining health functionings in particular, given the growing recognition of the psychological pathways between external social conditions and complex internal physiological processes, the distinc-tion between internal and combined capabilities may need to be less emphasized. In any case, for a person to have a certain level of CH, all four components – personal features/needs, behaviours, surrounding social and physical conditions – must be capable of coming together to create practical possibility to achieve each CHC up to or above the specified thresholds. The differential distribution patterns or asymmetrical achievements of the CH across individuals can be explained by the diversity in how individuals are uniquely 'constructed and situated'; how each individual faces different biology, physical and social conditions, and abilities to 'convert' these factors into beings and doings.

Structure and causal model of CH

An individual's CH should be understood to be dynamic. Most often, the CA literature presents a capability as a static attribute of a person, or as a simple unidirectional process or vector moving from capability to functioning achievement. In contrast, a person's over-arching CH or a particular CHC may be more accurately understood as a dynamic and iterative system made up of the four causal components of individual endowments, conversion skills, extant physical conditions and surrounding social conditions. At any given moment and over the life course, each of the ten capabilities and the over-arching CH is continually in flux, being shaped by dynamic processes underlying each causal component. Processes occurring at various levels ranging from biological processes at the sub-molecular level within the person (endowment) to the political and economic processes at the national and global level (physical and social conditions) constantly influence the capabilities of individuals. The relative influence of each causal component on a person's CH is specific to each individual and constantly changing over the life course. That is, national economic policies may constrain the CH of one individual as much or even more than the constraints produced by genetic endowment in another. And the individual's conversion skills and volitional choices affecting functioning achievements may expand or contract at different points in her lifetime.

Acknowledging the dynamicity and differences in causal components across individuals and the fact that the CH is ever-changing over the life course brings to the forefront the need to consider in more detail the concept of thresholds. A minimal standard of dignity is profoundly helpful because it provides a metric for comparing capabilities across individuals and over time. But in fact, identifying a single standard over the life course of one individual or across different individuals of the same or different ages, sexes, economic positions, abilities, talents, ambitions, and so forth is a daunting endeavour. The theoretical idea of a common standard is useful, but practically it has multiple dimensions (Sen, 1998b, 1998a).

Nussbaum provides a more detailed argument that the respect for the equal moral worth or ensuring minimal dignity of individuals entails 'supporting' or 'providing' threshold levels of each CHC. Entitlements to such social support or provision are not to the achievement itself, most often, but to the social bases of each capability (Nussbaum, 2000b, pp. 81–82). So far, Nussbaum only provides various examples of possible social bases of particular CHCs such as adequate nutrition, education of the faculties, protection of bodily integrity, and so forth (Nussbaum, 2006, p. 278). Her version of the CA has not posited a model of causation of CHCs, and the identification of the breadth of social bases, along with the exact levels of each CHC, are underdescribed or deferred to a later stage and expertise of various professionals. Such openness is partly due to the need for public deliberation and engendering the possibility of achieving global overlapping consensus on the list (Nussbaum, 2006, pp. 291–295). Though such openness to public deliberation is necessary, there is still much theoretical work to be done to integrate the concept of CHCs into a coherent conception of health, and theories of health causation and distribution.

The present argument for the CH pursues the line that the entitlement to each capability should be understood as the entitlement to the social bases of each causal component. And providing or supporting threshold levels of CH entails social action through influencing the social bases of the causal components of each capability. That is, protecting, promoting or restoring the CH of individuals to adequate levels is realized through the possible and justifiable interventions into personal features/needs, conversion skills, external physical conditions and surrounding social conditions.

Furthermore, the range of agents with obligations to protect, promote or restore the CH of individuals to the specified level, and the extent of their obligations will depend on how they stand in relation to the causes, consequences and distribution patterns of CH achievements and failures. For example, Onora O'Neill has written on the need to expand the breadth of relevant agents and obligations in light of individuals living where there are failed nation-states and where health threats cross national borders (O'Neill, 2002b, 2004b, 2004a). Thomas Pogge's recent arguments for negative, positive and intermediate duties may also be useful for mapping obligations of agents in relation to the causes, consequences, and distribution patterns of CH (Pogge, 1989, 2001, 2002b).

The argument for a sufficient level of CH does not in fact, produce an easy or single, uniform rule. Minimal dignity will be commensurate with different levels across each of the ten CHCs. Even then, the breadth of social bases, and the extent of justifiable intervention into those social bases of different causal components of each CHC will vary across persons. For any society, ensuring the CH of citizens means the assessment of the multiple dimensions of causes, consequences and distribution patterns of CH achievements and failures. The response will require varied actions to protect, promote or restore the CH of individuals to sufficient levels.

In contrast, the prevalent discussions on possible justice claims related to health often quickly turn to the distribution of healthcare. Sometimes, they extend to the provision of 'public health' goods such as sanitation, potable water, food safety, and so forth (Daniels, 1985; Kass, 2001, 2004). However, in the context of rich countries where clinical healthcare and public health goods and services are abundantly available, it is perhaps more readily apparent than in poor countries that avoiding premature mortality and impairments requires having control over one's body and behaviour as well as material goods such as healthcare. For example, when considering the spread of HIV/AIDS it becomes easy to see that in the absence of an HIV vaccine, avoiding infection requires having control over one's body and behaviour over the entire life course. Prior to global experience with HIV/AIDS and the women's health movement, it was commonplace to think that healthcare is necessary and sufficient to address health concerns.

Now, in the face of new and resurgent infectious diseases and research findings on social position and chronic impairments, it is more readily acknowledged that over the life course, and in different physical and social environments, commodities and 'autonomy' or 'agency' can be crucially important. For example, the ability to secure food directly becomes much more important as one gets older than when one is an infant being cared for by another person. Or, a person who has full access to clinical care may still need refuge away from physical abuse at home.

Such examples show that the focus only on goods, whether food, clinical care or something else, would only protect health functionings during some of the time periods in the life course. Individuals require autonomy and agency both to ward off avoidable physical threats as well as to seek out resources to achieve, maintain, protect and restore their own physical and mental functionings. This need for a mix of material goods and supportive social conditions for autonomy is reflected in the four components of the causal model of the CH.

Autonomy can be thought of as part of conversion skills component of the CH.

The importance of a person's abilities to act in addressing health concerns can also be shown in the Senian vector-idea of a capability. When a well-being functioning such as achieving internal immunity from a vaccine is not possible, then agency functionings become much more important in the protection of health functionings and indeed, all other capabilities. That is, for example, if direct beneficial immunity through a vaccine cannot be induced then abilities to be vigilant against exposure to infection become more important. Even when a vaccine is available, agency functionings can still be important in order to identify its availability and in procuring it. Perspectives which focus only on producing well-being functionings such as immunity through 'vertical-health programmes' or other healthcare goods aim to bypass inadequacies in agency functionings/conversion skills. The causal components of conversion skills, physical environment, and social conditions are thought to be 'distal factors' of health functionings that are outside the purview of health sector interventions.

It has been repeatedly argued that the needs for different types and amounts of commodities will vary across individuals, and over the life course. And the abilities to convert commodities into health functionings will also vary across individuals and over the life course. Not only can internal biological processes require different amounts of the same commodity among two individuals, they may also differ in their immediate abilities to reach for, ingest, apply or inject the commodity. This amounts to a difference in converting available resources into functionings. Importantly, individuals may also directly suffer from the provision of a standard amount or type of good when their particular individual needs and conversion skills are not sufficiently taken into account. It is quite common for public health policies applying a maximization approach to improving health achievements to accept that some individuals will suffer negative consequences from being provided with a standard public health good. For example, government programmes which promote or require the use of particular contraceptives without taking into account the unique needs of individuals may induce temporary or life-threatening consequences. When that occurs, the justification that the benefits to many outweigh the burden of the few shows that the individuals that suffer have not been treated as their own ends, or as a bearer of equal moral claims to a CH and equal dignity.

The maintenance and protection of CHCs of individuals in different places and times requires addressing threats in the environment that cannot be undertaken by a single individual or small group. That is, the required capacity to ensure the CH may be greater than that of any single individual. And, protecting individuals against certain kinds of health threats sometimes requires the social provision of protection for all individuals. Maintaining a safe water supply, immunizing schoolchildren and engaging in epidemiological research are some examples of the social provision of public goods aimed to ensure the capability to achieve health functionings of groups of individuals. And in certain places and times, protections of health functionings may require direct inducement of certain biological functionings such as producing herd immunity to particular infectious organisms through vaccinations. Protecting the capabilities of people through the provision of public goods can be seen as realizing 'passive' agency achievements of individuals (Pettit, 2001; Sen, 2001c).

CH and claims for research

If the causal pathway to the functioning, or the method of avoiding an impairment is not fully known, the claim to the social bases can entail claims to further research. How? Because social justice aims for the sufficiency and equity of capabilities among individuals. When individuals are constrained by impairments that cannot be mitigated or prevented, they are constrained from pursuing the beings and doings of a richer human life. In Nussbaum's conception, they are being denied a fully human life. In Frances Kamm's words, they are restricted from fully experiencing and enjoying life's experiential goods (Kamm, 1993).

Moreover, inequalities in CH across individuals unavoidably results in inequalities in many other capabilities or areas of life. Health capability and functionings determine the worth of other human capabilities. While respect for equal dignity would point to addressing avoidable causes of inequality in the CH, the value to a human being of having all the basic capabilities, and preserving the worth of all capabilities, drives the scientific research into unknown causes or how to mitigate impairments which currently have no treatment. It is this value of basic capabilities that drives social and medical science research into causes of impairments, and constitutes part of the social bases of capabilities.

One possible objection to this claim that all human beings have claim to CH, even if it is currently unknown what the cause or treatment might be, is that individuals cannot have entitlements or rights to something that is immediately not feasible. Ought implies can, and so someone ought to have a right implies that the individual can have the right. But if there are no known ways to bring the individual up to the threshold of being fully human, then they cannot have a right. Precisely in response to this kind of objections against rights, Sen has argued that individuals have meta-rights. According to Sen, 'a meta-right to something, x, can be defined as the right to have policies, p(x), that genuinely pursue the objective of making the right to x realizable' (Sen, 1984, p. 70).

So, if individuals have impairments caused by still unknown factors or no known methods of restoring capabilities exist, they can still have a meta-right that social institutions pursue policies that will help them realize their CH. This meta-right applies in contexts where social institutions cannot immediately ensure the rights of individuals because of the lack of resources as well as because of the lack of knowledge. Individuals can have a right to something as well as the right that social institutions must pursue policies, whether it is to do more research or improve social conditions, to realize the content of a right.

CH and social interdependency

The CH argument is centred on the conception of human dignity as partly arising out sociability or desire to live among other human beings in reciprocity and respect. However, it is important to recognize the vulnerability to impairments or premature mortality as a direct result of engaging in social cooperation. The moral relevance of the direct vulnerability to impairments from being among other human beings has been surprisingly under-considered by political philosophers and even bioethicists (Francis, 2005).

When one assumes away or excludes health issues in theorizing about basic principles of social justice, health threats which arise only and directly because of social cooperation are understandably going to become invisible. Yet, the threat of infectious diseases only arises when there are a sufficient number of other human beings around to sustain the propagation of the infectious organism. And, in such a case, the achievement, maintenance, protection and possible restoring of CH of an individual is unlikely to be fully achieved by the individual acting alone. The predominant focus on individual behaviour and volitional choices in dealing with vulnerability to infectious diseases fundamentally underplays the social bases of vulnerability to infectious diseases.

Additional vulnerability to impairments and mortality arising directly from social cooperation must be thought of as another 'burden' in distributing the benefits and burdens of social cooperation. The CH argument is able to recognize such vulnerability through the social conditions causal component. The CA does not erase inter-dependency.

Furthermore, Chapter 2 described the growing understanding of social determinants of health research. Social inequalities in the psychological experiences of individuals such as stress, social support networks, income inequality, discrimination and hopelessness produce differences in health capability. A life that is made up of few choices and which is lived in an unsupportive or unresponsive environment leads to the impairments of basic biological and psychological functionings. An organism that is stressed becomes vulnerable not only to a specific impairment but becomes generally more prone to injuries and accidents as well as to pathogenic organisms. So the individual's health capability is intrinsicly bound up with social relations; it is both created through as well as vulnerable to social relations. The CH as presented here is able to capture the social conditions, the conditions of mutual enterprise, affecting access to material resources and social conditions that in turn affect individual psychological experiences, which affect the abilities of individuals to carry out certain activities.

CH as 'mid-fare'

Some of the major alternative ethical approaches that do not focus on capabilities either recognize claims only to achieving certain mental states such as pleasure production or preference satisfaction, or eschew concern for mental states altogether and focus only on the provision of resources. The CA falls somewhere in between, as resources are necessary for realizing a capability, and the mental state of a person is both a source of information and also a locus of well-being for that individual. Though it is important to criticize theories that rely wholly on subjective mental states, it would be untenable to exclude completely mental states or functionings from an assessment of person's well-being, as they are valuable achievements in a human life. But welfare and resource theories suffer the problem of having *only* to consider welfare or resource holdings.

Once again, Nussbaum's cluster of CHCs proves useful for establishing the inter-dependency of capabilities and functionings, including psychological functionings. She identifies the capabilities of using senses, imagination, and thought; of being able to exercise emotions; of being able to form social associations, and importantly, of being able to use reason (Nussbaum, 2006, pp. 76–77). The CHCs reflect both physical functionings and psychological functionings; the 'objective' list of capabilities recognizes the importance of both resources and subjective welfare but targets capabilities.

CH as a 'cluster-right'

In fleshing out the entitlement to the CH, or to the cluster of CHCs, it is plausible and advantageous to argue that such an entitlement contains within it a multitude of claims, powers, privileges and immunities. The claim to the social bases of the CH is obviously broader than being just a 'positive' claim to things. It is easy in the first instance to outline an argument that the entitlement to the CH entails a positive claim to healthcare or other health-affecting goods. Yet, the claims for social support through social conditions can also be 'negative' claims against harmful physical events and social processes. Both positive and negative claims can be far-reaching and inter-related.

Moreover, the emphasis in the CA on having the freedom to choose among opportunities means not only having positive and negative claims but also powers, privileges and immunities. But which is the most important or relevant aspect will depend on the health-related issue at hand. And generally, more work needs to be done to map these various kinds of entitlements onto the diverse range of corresponding agents and their actions.

The CH, and indeed every capability, is really a cluster of iterative capabilities and functionings. The picture of a capability as being the opportunity of achieving a functioning which then is chosen to be achieved is a very simplified image that abstracts from complex processes underlying any single capability and functioning achievement. Nussbaum's advocacy of threshold levels of CHCs also gives the impression that a capability can be quantified and compared across individuals using a single metric. However, the causal model of capabilities put forward here shows that a single capability cannot be easily isolated from a cluster of inter-related capabilities and functionings, or easily distinguished as being a wholly internal or external capability.

Each capability is constantly in flux, being formed by the iterative and interactive processes involving personal features, conversion abilities, exposure to physical environment, social conditions and, importantly, the actual choices made by the individual. In light of this more complicated picture of a capability and its causal components, an entitlement to a capability, or more accurately, to the social bases of each of the causal components of a capability, should be understood as being a 'cluster-right'.

Judith Jarvis Thomson's identification of a 'cluster-right' is very useful to flesh out entitlements to any capability in the CA, and particularly in relation to the CH as advocated here. Thomson's cluster-right is a 'right that contains rights' (Thomson, 1990, pp. 54–56), in contrast with the classic or standard notion of a right as being a single claim with a corresponding duty-holder, Thomson's cluster-right can contain various combinations of claims, privileges, liberties, immunities and powers. As a result, not all rights involve corresponding duty holders.

Furthermore, equality or equity of a cluster-right across individuals, and even over a single life course, is indeed more difficult to evaluate than a simple claim-right, but it is not impossible or novel. In fact, Thomson argues many familiar rights such as the rights to life, liberty and property are more accurately understood as cluster-rights (Thomson, 1990, pp. 55, 272–293). There is frequent appraisal of these complex rights in many different societies, particularly in court-rooms and legal journals, which evinces that a cluster-right is a practicable concept.

The notion of a cluster-right is latent in various aspects of the CA literature. The Senian analytical device of a capability is described as having four vectors: well-being agency, well-being freedom, agency freedom and agency achievement. These four dimensions are said to describe plural dimensions of a capability. Continuing in that vein, one would expect that an entitlement to such a capability would be to all four vectors, and that claims to well-being and agency functioning would entail different kind of actions by various agents. For example, agency functionings can entail both freedoms from interference and also positive claims to goods necessary to act. And as Dan Brock argues, each of these four vectors can be thought as being made up even more indeterminate number of sub-vectors (Brock, 1995). Thus, articulating any sort of entitlement to a Senian capability would lead to an idea of an entitlement to a cluster of multi-dimensional claims. The range of well-being and agency freedoms and achievements would require various kinds of liberties, powers, privileges and immunities.

Thomson's argument for a cluster-right also supports Nussbaum's notion of CHCs by making plausible that different CHCs can each have unique thresholds, and that they do not have to be the same across individuals. The notion of a single threshold across individuals and across a lifetime was open to the criticism that it is impracticable or does not accurately reflect the causation of each CHC. With Thomson's cluster-right, each CHC and all the ten CHCs can be thought of as being plausible, despite giving rise to different sorts of claims across each of the ten CHCs, across individuals, and over the life course. So instead of there being a single metric and rule where a single point is considered sufficient, there is now a ruler in the shape of a branch with numerous rules with different possible points of sufficiency.

Indeed, Thomson's idea of cluster right, and its close approximation to a cluster of capabilities, initially motivated pursuing the concept of the CH as a meta-capability. Rather than a right to health being a claim to some single thing or a protection from a single thing, it was intuitively plausible to think of having the capability to be healthy as being made up of satisfying needs, having opportunities, powers, immunities, protections and so forth. And Nussbaum's ten CHCs, when more thoroughly considered, are not seen as being individually distinct, but as an inter-related cluster of basic capabilities. They are listed separately for the purposes of discussion, not in order to reflect their inherent independence. Thomson's cluster-right and Nussbaum's ten inter-related capabilities work well together. Not only does the notion of a cluster right apply to a single capability it also applies to the entire cluster of ten inter-related capabilities. The causal model of a capability that I have advanced and the idea of a cluster-right give the argument for ten CHCs more integrated and fleshed-out conceptual grounding. As a practical example, one can see in Jocelyn DeJong's research on capabilities and the reproductive health of poor women how protecting, promoting and restoring health involves various kinds of claims, powers, immunities and so forth (DeJong, 2006).

Kamm and capabilities

There is an alternative path to arriving at an ethical conception of the CH to that of Nussbaum's CHCs and notion of dignity, or from extending Nordenfelt's argument for achieving vital goals. For any person, being alive can be inherently valuable, while staying alive can also be crucially important to pursuing any possible conception of life plans. The moral force of such bland statements may become more apparent when death is seen in terms of the loss of the 'goods of life'. By goods of life Frances Kamm refers to such things as experiences, achievements, character, wisdom and relationships (Kamm, 1993). Death is a morally bad thing because it deprives individuals of experiential goods (deprivation), is a loss of goods for an already existing person (insult), and it forecloses any further possibilities for the person (extinction) (Kamm, 1993). She writes that if these kinds of losses happen from death after a normal lifespan, then a premature death must be an even more troublesome thing because it would be the loss of even more experiential goods than would have been lost after a normal lifespan.

Indeed, aside from dying with fewer experiential goods in absolute terms, the good of having the opportunity to choose among experiences, or what kind of life one wants to lead, is also lost. The CA highlights the importance of choice in a person's life, both in terms of having a breadth of meaningful choices as well as being the agent who chooses how one's life proceeds. Kamm seems to overlook choice as being a very important good of life unless she thinks it is subsumed under experiential goods.

Interestingly, Kamm's experiential goods can also be understood in terms of capabilities as they refer to beings and doings that human beings have reason to value. Death can be seen as a bad thing because it deprives people of experiencing various capabilities and functionings; it is a loss of previously held capabilities; and it forecloses acquiring any further capabilities. There is also again, value in being able to choose which capabilities to pursue and therefore, death would also be the loss of the good of being able to choose among capabilities. Pursuing this line of thought, a set of basic capabilities and functionings could be identified that would allow a person to pursue the beings and doings one has reason to value, or in Kamm's terms, the goods of life.

Seen as the essential or basic capabilities and functioning that make all other capabilities possible, the CH is valuable because it determines the real 'worth' of all other capabilities of pursuing one's life plans. At the same time, physical and mental impairments can significantly constrain the effective opportunities to pursue the goods of life. Paralleling the effects of death on the goods of life and capabilities, so too can impairments, which are less final than death, deprive individuals of experiencing capabilities, lead to the loss of existing capabilities and foreclose certain other capabilities. Death and impairments simply belong on a spectrum of constraints that restrict the goods of life.

While Kamm's analysis can give structure and coherence to some of our moral intuitions regarding death and impairments, she does not seem to identify what moral claims human beings have to such experiential goods, or what the social response should be to losses of such goods. As I have argued, we can view capabilities and choosing capabilities and functionings as goods of life. And death and impairments can indeed lead to various kinds of losses of capabilities. But why capabilities are morally important, and what claims human beings have to their capabilities must also be identified and justified. Labelling them goods of life does not express sufficiently their centrality or value in the lives of human beings. Such questions regarding claims and justification may be more productively answered within broader frameworks of theories of social justice. Thus, it is a significant achievement that Nussbaum has presented an accessible, freestanding theory of the good; what Kamm might refer to as the goods of life. Nussbaum identifies some central capabilities, or goods of life, that reflect the dignity of the human being. And she identifies that such a conception of dignity exerts claims or entitlements for social support.

Why the CH

Aside from avoiding the shortcomings of resourcist or welfarist approaches, the entitlement to the CH also expands the traditional scope of health claims. The scope of the entitlement to the CH includes protections against all the social bases of impairments and mortality. In contrast, even the most committed advocate of the CA currently takes as given existing disease categories and evidentiary power of available statistics on the prevalence of morbidity and mortality. Theorists who understand health claims as being only those arising in the clinical setting, or having to do just with disease, are blind to many other sources of health claims.

Such an understanding comes from the pervasive and incoherent notion of disease in the medical sciences. The concepts of disease, and health as the absence of disease, must be jettisoned as our knowledge of the causes of impairments and mortality has outstripped their value. As the causal model of the CH argues, the breadth of components including personal features/needs, conversion skills, exposures to physical environment and social conditions produce health capability and have moral relevance.

A sufficient social response to health capability constraints must evaluate the social bases of all the causal components. For example, the poor nutrition of girls and women in developing countries is hardly ever considered within a medical setting, and is even less likely a topic for health policy or bioethics. The distribution of food within the household in resource-poor settings has been shown to be a function of the gender of individuals. Yet, the consideration of the social conditions within and outside the household affecting gender and consequent access to nutrition is rarely, if ever, part of health policy. As malnutrition is not due to disease, or even when it does lead to disease, the social determinants are still left unaddressed. For both instrumental and ethical reasons, there needs to be a reorientation of health concerns away from the narrow focus on disease to the CH. An entitlement to the CH would be able to recognize the nutritional deprivation of females as a health issue, be able to identify the differing causal factors, and provide the moral force to mitigate the social bases of such nutritional deprivation.

Objections

A possible objection to this conception of the CH is that it is too expansive. Even after agreement that there is a claim to a capability to be healthy, there may be reticence in defining health as being more than 'within the skin' assessment of physiological functionings. In this view, healthcare is meant to address the body not the social environment. If that is what clinical medical care aims to do, then fine. But the compulsion to whittle down the components of a CH to some 'core' biological, statistically normal, 'species typical', or perhaps, culturally relative capabilities and functionings should be resisted from the start. Human health viewed as a capability and grounded in the respect for freedoms, human dignity and equal moral worth has more conceptual coherence and is more robust in evaluating the empirical aspects of human mortality and impairments than the commonplace understanding of health as the absence of disease. And it is also more contained than the definition of health as total individual and social well-being.

The absence of disease model, despite being the background conception in contemporary health sciences, relies on a notion of statistical frequency that is not 'value-free' as is claimed and exhibits many conceptual defects in theory and practice. I discussed some of these in Chapter 1. And the total well-being notion is grounded in a crude perfectionist account of human life, and can be criticized for being a purely utopian ideal (Lafaille and Fulder, 1993). In contrast to either of these options, a coherent conception of human health can be plausibly conceived as being able to achieve vital goals, or a cluster of basic capabilities and functionings that constitute a life of activity and opportunity worthy of the dignity of the human being in the modern world.

Nussbaum's CHCs or conception of minimal human dignity provides a defensible set of such basic activities and opportunities as well as limits the conception of the CH from becoming too expansive such as the notion of health as complete physical, mental and social well-being. Some might try to assert that because Nussbaum has identified bodily health as the second capability, there is some redundancy in saying that all ten capabilities make up health capability. The idea of a meta-capability to achieve CHCs can include the narrow focus on disease and impairments of biological functionings while preserving the demarcation between health and complete well-being. The extant health capability in Nussbaum's list can be seen as referring to biological functioning, while all the basic capabilities put together refer to health. This conception of health is also then less expansive than total wellbeing. And, the argument for the meta-capability makes a distinction between the abilities and actual achievements of well-being so that it is not aiming to induce various functionings socially. To be healthy is to have a sufficient level of capabilities of pursuing life plans in contemporary global society that is commensurate with equal human dignity.

Conclusion

On the one hand, the present argument for the CH provides a coherent conceptual vehicle for evaluating the descriptive aspects of the determinants, consequences, persistence and distribution of human impairments and mortality. On the other hand, the moral, pre-political entitlement to the social basis of a CH is also more coherent and justifiable than the hitherto received view of health claims as either claims to healthcare resources or health welfare (subjective and objective) achievements. Part of the weakness of both resource and welfare health entitlements are that they are significantly qualified by a range of limitations, including the emphasis on individual volitional choices and behaviour, social borders and the amount of local resources, current limits on scientific knowledge and technology, the requirements of other social goals, and the morality of luck. As such, the weaknesses of the arguments for entitlements to healthcare or health achievements closely parallel the weaknesses of the more general arguments for distributing resources or welfare in pursuing social justice. The next chapter reviews how resource and welfare theories handle health claims, reviews their weaknesses, and argues that the CH can do better than them in many respects.

Part III

5

Alternative Approaches

In this chapter I consider alternative ethical approaches to health claims to those that focus on capabilities. First, I will review the health equity principles initially articulated by Margaret Whitehead and which have significantly influenced public health, social epidemiology and health policy. Then, I will review the health and human rights approach advocated by Jonathan Mann and colleagues and evaluate its contributions to discussions about health and justice. The remaining part of the chapter will consider how health claims are handled by more general ethical approaches to social justice and which concentrate on the distribution of welfare or resources. I give detailed attention to Norman Daniels' argument for health justice, as he has recently been writing that his extension of Rawls' theory and subsequent amendments makes it virtually similar to the capabilities approach. Finally, while I do not think it is a fully fledged theory of justice, I also discuss a good version of a luck egalitarian argument related to health justice. Despite being a useful exercise in clarifying the similarities and differences, I conclude that the capabilities approach to health justice is still the more coherent and less morally erroneous approach.

In Chapter 3 I briefly contrasted the CA with resourcist and welfarist/utilitarian approaches by discussing how the CA was initially developed in reaction to these approaches. The differences are brought into greater relief here through focusing in particular on how they handle health-related claims. As with Chapter 3, the present discussion is not meant to be comprehensive but aims to highlight the salient differences and to argue further for how the CH argument does better in some ways than the competing ethical approaches in evaluating and responding to human health concerns. As I said in the Introduction, one can list a large number of other approaches to social justice such as libertarianism, feminism, communitarianism, republicanism, multiculturalism and so forth. And it is indeed possible to apply a range of these different ethical approaches to health claims (Childress et al., 2002; Roberts and Reich, 2002). I have chosen five for closer examination. The reason for focusing on these five approaches is that they are the most recognizable and influential approaches in real-world health policy and in the nascent theoretical deliberations about health and social justice. The comparison of the CA and CH with other approaches awaits further enquiry.

Health equity principles

Over the past twenty years or so, the public concern for the persistence of inequalities in health outcomes across social and geographical groups in industrialized countries as well as concern about the persistence of high prevalence of preventable mortality and impairments in poor countries have been brought together under the umbrella term 'health equity' (Whitehead, 1990; Evans et al., 2001; Braveman and Gruskin, 2003; Braveman, 2006). In order to motivate social action to address health inequalities within and across countries, and appropriately target social action, it is argued that ethical values compel decreasing 'health inequities' across social groups. 'Inequities' is meant to be a moral and ethical term in contrast to 'inequalities' which is seen as term referring to value-free observable differences. Because all health impairments, including the ultimate impairment of death, are not necessarily morally troubling, to identify which subset of all impairments or inequalities qualify as inequities that require a response as a matter of social justice, three criteria in the form of a decision tree have been put forward (Whitehead, 1990). A health difference or inequality becomes a health inequity when it is deemed to be (a) avoidable, (b) unnecessary, and (c) unfair or unjust. Society is said to be morally obligated to act to prevent and mitigate the health impairments that remain after applying the three-tier filter (Whitehead, 1990; Whitehead, 1992; Evans et al., 2001).

Though it has admirable intent, and has had great influence in motivating public policy and an international movement for promoting health equity, there are a number of conceptual weaknesses in the three-pronged health equity approach. Whitehead offers a summary of the reasoning as, 'Equity in health implies that ideally everyone should have a fair opportunity to attain their full health potential and, more pragmatically, that no one should be disadvantaged from achieving this potential, if it can be avoided' (Whitehead, 1990, p. 7). Furthermore, she writes that based on this definition of health equity the aim of policy should be, '. . . to reduce or eliminate those [health differences] which result from factors which are considered to be both avoidable and unfair' (Whitehead, 1990, p. 7).

Despite the more detailed articulation of 'equity in health' and the aim of policy, there still remains a lack of clarity about the scope and target of moral concern and action, especially if it is meant to be applied across all countries. The most prominent weakness is the overarching vagueness about whether the moral concern over 'health differences' is related to the distribution patterns of health constraints – seen in terms of relative health differences between social groups – or for other dimensions, such as the absolute levels of health functionings and potential, for the types of causes, for the consequences, the extant possibilities of mitigation, or for all of these aspects.

In the first instance, are we worried primarily about relative health inequalities between groups, or that some groups have poor health and are not achieving what they could, evidenced by what other groups are achieving? And secondly, are we worried about inter-group inequalities and inter-individual inequalities, or just group inequalities, or group inequalities because of our concern for individuals within them? These questions about whether our moral concern in health equity is for equality or *priority* and whether concern is for groups or individuals, or both, are crucially important to answer as they determine all the reasoning that follows (Parfit, 1997; Murray et al., 1999b; Braveman et al., 2000; Gakidou et al., 2000; Braveman et al., 2001).

Aside from this general ambiguity about inequality of what, there is a lack of clarity at each step of the decision tree. At the first decision level, making the first cut between what is avoidable and unavoidable, there is no distinction between whether a health difference should be considered as being unavoidable because of the lack of resources or because there is no extant epidemiological knowledge about aetiology, control or treatment. For example, impairments related to ageing can be seen either as being inevitable or that we do not know how to prevent or control them. And both limitations in resources and knowledge can make a health constraint, including the ultimate constraint of death, unavoidable at a point in time or given location. However, given that health equity advocates are greatly concerned with extreme global health disparities, it would take the bite out of the approach if limits on resources available locally were allowed to determine what is avoidable. Because limited financial resources and institutional capacities are obvious and significant reasons why health constraints persist in many poor countries, most of the health disparities would become unavoidable and thus could not be identified as inequities and socially actionable.

At the same time, if limited local resources and institutional capacities are not factors we should use in determining whether a health constraint is avoidable, then it is unclear who the agent is who is supposed to be compelled to act by the moral force of this framework in such circumstances. If local institutions cannot act because they lack resources, who is obligated by these principles to remedy the inequity by satisfying the local resource needs or stand in for the absent institutional capacities?

A different set of implications follow when existing medical or scientific knowledge determines whether a health constraint is avoidable or not. First, depending wholly on the expertise of epidemiologists to determine which constraint is avoidable or not means taking as given existing disease categories and their underlying epidemiology. This would absolve any social obligations from fairness or justice to assist individuals with impairments and causes of mortality that are not currently recognized by 'Western medicine' such as those listed in the ICD-10 (World Health Organization, 2007).[1]

Second, because the criterion of 'avoidable' relies first and foremost on scientific knowledge of aetiology, control and prevention, it expresses full confidence in the epistemology, coherence and ethics of the practice of epidemiology. Yet, the history of research scientists' engagement with health affairs such as women's reproductive health or HIV/AIDS should caution against such wholehearted confidence in epidemiology's objective pursuit of scientific knowledge and practice (Reid, 1992; Angell, 1993; Epstein, 1996). And such deference does not seem to appreciate to what extent epidemiology is itself a social product and uses particular cultural conceptions of person, place and time (Trostle, 2004; Venkatapuram, 2006).

Third, as I discussed in Chapter 2, the current paradigm in epidemiology is limited in a number of ways that obscures and misclassifies the causes, distribution and possible social remedies of health impairments. Fourth, because the criterion of 'justice and fairness' is the last step, those health constraints and their disparities that become classified as unavoidable or 'necessary' by the first two steps fall outside the scope of ethics and justice. That is, no claims from justice are available to individuals who experience unavoidable or 'necessary' impairments and mortality. Simply put, considering justice and fairness last means that the expertise of epidemiologists is allowed to define the scope and content of ethics rather than ethics driving the purpose and scope of the instrumental science of epidemiology (Marmot, 1976; Khushf, 1987; Weed, 1996; Weed and McKeown, 1998, 2001; Venkatapuram and Marmot, 2009).

Even if we were to accept justice and fairness as the last consideration, the health equity approach expresses no clear commitment to a particular conception of justice or fairness. There are references to human rights, and oblique references to Rawlsian social justice, and to the capabilities approach (Ostlin and Diderichsen, 2001; Peter and Evans, 2001; Anand, 2002; Braveman and Gruskin, 2003). It is also important to note that despite the use of human rights rhetoric by health equity advocates, the three-pronged view is actually unsympathetic to rights. The view expresses a particular form of utilitarianism – rule utilitarianism – where the underlying argument is that the state of the world would be much better overall (i.e. more healthy) if certain human rights, such as access to a minimum package of healthcare goods and services, were protected, provided or promoted.

The protection of rights is invoked here as part of a purely consequentialist view rather than expressing deontological ethics.[2] Health equity advocates would probably have great difficulty navigating the conflict between rights and unlikely to side with rights in the classic conflict between individual rights and increasing overall social benefit. Decreasing the magnitude of health differences or inequities is likely to have priority over respecting individual rights. As the current health equity discussions are largely focused on alleviating the stark aggregate health inequalities across social groups or geographic populations, what rights or claims individuals have under a health equity regime is unclear.

This three-tiered approach to responding to health constraints is clearly an exercise in applied philosophy. It seeks to apply ethical principles to existing institutions and practices, particularly in the clinical and public health sciences. Ethicists are often fond of saying that 'ought implies can' and thus, it seems understandable to initiate a health equity analysis with existing health institutions and their capacities, particularly taking epidemiological science as it is. But the shortcomings of this intuitive or deductive method of applied philosophy, of identifying ethical principles from meta-analysis of literature and practice, are also clear in this situation.

Considering the aetiology of an impairment or health difference as being avoidable or not prior to what justice requires evidences a view that health is foremost a phenomenon of nature, a 'natural good', to which social institutions must respond. Such a view is untenable given our growing recognition of the social production of determinants of impairments and mortality within and across societies. Social interactions have not only improved human longevity and functioning, but also produce impairments, premature mortality and their distribution. Considerations of justice, or the principles that govern the actions of individuals and social institutions, cannot be secondary to the factors of 'human nature' but must be integrated with it. Giving priority to scientific knowledge about causation and distribution of disease in determining the scope of fairness and justice gives too much deference to science.

Perhaps the most ethically troubling part of the three-pronged criteria is how it deals with individuals who have unavoidable or necessary impairments. The social response to individuals who are vulnerable to or experience unavoidable or necessary impairments or mortality (i.e. collateral damage) cannot just be silence, nor are they a matter for charity (Kittay, 1997; Nussbaum, 2006; Wasserman, 2006). Within the health equity framework they are literally pushed outside the margins of moral concern. Respect for their equal moral worth has to be recognized and accounted for somewhere. And, the notion that some mortality or impairments are necessary is profoundly problematic, requiring extraordinary justification as a matter of justice, and cannot be presupposed to be acceptable as is done here.

Though the health equity principles and movement are commendable for drawing on ethics to motivate greater social action addressing health inequalities, it is unfortunately insufficient as an ethical framework. Relying on the capacity of existing institutions, even if it is scientific expertise, precludes the comprehensive ethical evaluation of the causes, persistence, levels, variable consequences and distribution patterns of health constraints as well as possible social remedies. All of these dimensions of human health, and probably many more, have moral relevance.

The question of which impairment or mortality is unjust or unfair across individuals and groups – because of its causes, consequences, distribution, or possibility of remedy – must precede considering what our current social institutions are capable of addressing. If the right social institutions or capacities do not currently exist to address unjust or unfair health constraints, then our ethics should compel us to create such institutions and capacities.[3] Given what we already know about the healthcare and broader social determinants of health and health inequalities, substantial improvements in health and health inequalities will require significant social change, resources, inter-sectoral government policies, social participation and so forth. The ethical evaluation of health and health inequalities at the population level requires more than a casuistic or ad-hoc set of principles. It requires that we put health at the centre of our theorizing about social justice and see what sort of guidance that provides.

Health and human rights

Starting in the mid to late 1980s, health advocates began increasingly to draw on the principles and mechanisms of international human rights law because of a series of events. Some advocates were involved in the international women's health movement, some worked in humanitarian emergencies, and others were addressing the global spread of HIV and AIDS. In all of these cases, the health issues cut across countries where there was no functioning state. There was a need to find supra-national mechanisms to affect national policy or address the needs of those who had no government. In the first instance, human rights law offered protection to human beings against oppressive government actions. But the health and human rights approach evolved from there to be much broader. The idea was that international human rights law taken as a whole, rather than selectively prioritizing one covenant over another, offers both rights to healthcare and rights to the social and material conditions for good health. This framework was put forward by Jonathan Mann and colleagues in the first issue of the *Journal of Health and Human Rights* in 1994 (Mann et al., 1994). Central to their 'health and human rights framework' hypothesis was the idea that 'the promotion and protection of human rights and promotion and protection of health are fundamentally linked'.

It was clear by the early 1990s in light of the way HIV/AIDS was being dealt with in most countries that public health programmes can negatively affect human rights, and that human rights violations can have negative health effects. For example, public health programmes were often very coercive and such programmes drove people underground, making the spread of infections much worse. Mann and colleagues transformed the conflict between a public health policy perspective and a human rights perspective into a hypothesis that a society which realizes the full breadth of human rights would produce healthier individuals and populations. Health programmes, whether public health or clinical, which were in line with human rights law would lead to better health outcomes, and the respect for all human rights would create conditions for individuals to be healthier. It was a vision of health and the good society.

One noteworthy aspect of the Mann hypothesis is that it leads to conceptualizing human rights law as components of an epidemiological model of causation and distribution of health. This is illustrated in that initial article in the discussion on possible ways of testing the hypothesis. They wrote: 'For example, health professionals could consider using the International Bill of Human Rights as a coherent guide for assessing health status of individuals or populations; the extent to which human rights are realized may represent a better and more comprehensive index of well-being than traditional health status indicators' (Mann et al., 1994).

While it was a groundbreaking contribution to overlay human rights law onto an analysis of the causes, distribution and social responses to health issues, the consequent substitution of human rights law for the actual causes in a model of causation and distribution of health is problematic, and the source of many disagreements and ill feelings today. For example, the distinction between the lack of sutures and the lack of the right to sutures in explaining the cause of maternal mortality is profound in many respects and should not be glossed over.

The observation of the lack of sutures in the causes of maternal mortality comes prior to reasoning that there should be a right to sutures. Some human rights advocates want to assert that it is the violation of the right to sutures which causes maternal mortality. When it is asserted that the lack of a right to something is the cause of ill-health and mortality, the distinction between the causal role and importance of that something, and the right to that something collapses. Moreover, it creates confusion as to what is a human right. Human rights are not natural things but are ethical assertions about claims, privileges, liberties, immunities and powers in relation to various human capabilities, including indirectly via material things. Attempting to emphasize the importance of human rights by casting them as direct causal components of a model of causation and distribution of ill-health and mortality produces unnecessary and avoidable misunderstandings. Furthermore, it undermines the important scientific analysis of causal pathways and distribution of impairments and opens the analysis to being dismissed as conceptually incoherent. Lastly, such an analysis potentially alienates social and natural science researchers who can be valuable allies in the effort to advance health equity. The health and human rights framework can be very powerful indeed, if it supplements rather than attempt to substitute the analysis of the multiple dimensions of impairments and mortality.

Health rights

But the health and human rights approach that Mann advanced is not the only way health and the ethical idea of rights have come together. The idea of rights has seeped into political discourse around the world. Whether expressed as human rights, civil rights, women's rights, minority rights, children's rights and so forth, rights language is used to articulate particular human interests as basic and urgent. Rights language further expresses that such interests require special attention from national governments and increasingly, foreign governments and international civil society. It is an important development in the global proliferation of the idea of rights that rights language is being used to articulate interests of people in relation to disease, disability and premature mortality ('health rights').

In the United States, for example, limitations on the type and amount of healthcare provided to patients determined by health insurance companies as well as the high price of pharmaceuticals has resulted in a public outcry. The American public is calling for the protection of health interests of people through greater government regulation of insurance and pharmaceutical companies. At the same time, there has been a re-emergence of the call for the government to guarantee every citizen access to some level of healthcare, and has achieved some success. On the other hand, in many of the world's poor countries, social movements seeking to improve the health of girls and women or to combat the HIV/AIDS epidemic have explicitly used rights language to make claims on public resources that are widely acknowledged as being severely limited.

'Health rights' properly constructed and justified can offer valid justification for substantive claims to public resources and as such, constrain the increasing influence of cost-effective analysis in the planning and evaluation of health programmes. A coherent understanding of 'health rights' can also offer a complementary framework to the economic, epidemiological and demographic analysis of the determinants, levels, consequences and responses to preventable morbidity and mortality. While these two contributions could be significant on their own, 'health rights' also have the more profound potential to clarify, reaffirm or indeed, redefine the fundamental purposes and duties of the state as well as the moral obligations of persons across national borders.

However, the present 'health rights' discourse is unlikely to yield such fruits. The possible benefits are largely being deferred due to confusing political and moral rhetoric of rights that superficially cuts across or completely ignores longstanding discussions. The language of 'health rights' is being used in both rich and poor countries opportunistically, as an instrumental means to achieve immediate policy outcomes while wholly side-stepping fundamental conceptual gaps within and between the ideas of rights, health and (global) justice. This is partly the reason why health economists and health policy-makers shun the idea of rights. If 'health rights' are to be understood as something more ethically significant than strong 'interests' or 'preferences' of various groups seeking to manipulate the health policy-making process or hoard limited resources, more rigorous and careful attempts to clarify and justify such rights are desperately needed.

Indeed, because the ability to stay alive and to function physically and mentally are fundamental requirements to pursuing a good life, 'health rights' advocates perhaps, more than any other rights advocates, carry the burden of showing how the idea of rights can be coherent in the context of limited resources. They are also burdened with tackling head on the embarrassing blind-spot in the philosophy of liberalism which gives pride of place to the protection of basic, individual rights that enable a person to pursue a good life, but nevertheless, the philosophy does not seem to identify any moral obligations across national borders to assist people being denied such rights (Beitz, 1975; O'Neill, 1993; Shapiro and Brilmayer, 1999).

The form, content and justification of the various 'health rights' arguments in rich and poor countries can be organized into four categories. The first category includes claims to disease and disability specific responses (e.g. research, drugs, medical services, legal protections, etc.) expressed as rights made by and on behalf of individuals affected by disease and disability (e.g. HIV infection, haemophilia, physical disability, reproductive morbidity, etc.). The second category includes claims to various packages of health-affecting goods and services (e.g. basic healthcare, clean water, adequate sanitation, etc.) based on rights already articulated in national and human rights law. The difference between these two categories is sometimes obfuscated when claims to disease and disability-specific responses are justified as being derived from rights established in national and international human rights law. The third category of arguments is indirect as it seeks the protection of a range of rights established in national and international law which are empirically shown to have effects on the health of persons. For example, the right to freedom of expression is shown to be instrumental in preventing and responding to famines, prevention of HIV infections, or improving reproductive and sexual health.

At the same time, in the related discipline of political philosophy, there has been a growing interest in health and social justice under-stood as the examination of the relationships between justice, equality and the health of persons and populations. Thus, the fourth category includes rights arguments with respect to the health interests of persons that are derived from various foundational theories and principles of justice. That is to say, the rights discussed here are derived from theo-ries of justice and moral reasoning, rather than starting from legal instruments.

For example, Norman Daniels argues, based on Rawls' theory of justice as fairness that a just society requires that people have the equality of opportunity to achieve offices of social advantage and, as being healthy is a necessary and vital component of having such equal opportunity, adequate healthcare should be guaranteed to every person. Therefore, individuals have a right to healthcare because a just society ensures equality of opportunity, and health is an impor-tant part of someone's equality of opportunity (Daniels, 1985). Utili-tarians might say that all individuals have a right to have their preferences counted in the determination of the policy which will lead to the greatest utility. And, of course, I have been arguing in this book that every human being has an entitlement or right to the capability to be healthy based on the value of freedom and respect for equal dignity.

This is not the place to review in detail all the different practical ways rights are used in relation to health, their coherence, or various issues in the health and human rights approach. What I wanted to do was present how rights, which are ethical ideas, have been used in relation to health claims so far. The success of the rights approaches, whether at the national or at the international level, has been enor-mous. But from a philosophical perspective, human rights or any other rights have to be grounded in some general ethical theory or approach. We cannot justify rights by pointing to legal instruments. Indeed, is it not ethical reasoning that produced certain values which then became enshrined as various rights in human rights law in the first place? Because ethical reasoning produces rights, we have to dig deeper to get right the ethical reasoning about individuals and their health claims. If we can achieve that, then it will not be as easy to dismiss the human right to health as incoherent or just emotional rhetoric to advocate for vested interests. That is what this book has been aiming to do. By providing a coherent concept of health as capability, a theory of causation and distribution of health capability, and making health part of the conversation about first principles of social organization, I have attempted to build a human right to the capability to be healthy from first principles.

Welfare theories and health

As I said in Chapter 3, which reviewed the capabilities approach, there are seen to be three main schools in the debates about distributive justice. As Elizabeth Anderson succinctly states, all theories of distributive justice have a metric and rule (Anderson, 2010, p. 81). They identify what the object is that is relevant to justice, the metric, and how to distribute it, the rule. The three major alternatives are resources, welfare or capabilities. In contrast to the diversity of entitlements encompassed by a cluster-right that is the CH, and the multiple dimensions of causes, consequences, persistence, levels and distribution, possible social responses and the varied duties to protect, promote and restore the CH, a welfarist approach to health would probably focus just on maximizing a single metric of health across individuals. And this health metric would be related to utility, some mental characteristic, such as pleasure, happiness, satisfaction or desire related to physical and mental functionings. In its simplest form, such a metric could be 'mortality cases averted'; there would be more utility from people living than if they were dead.

But how do we measure utility related to states of being that have to do with health? That is to say, how do we measure utility in relation to states of being in between fully functioning and complete death? Such a health measurement is seen to be necessary in at least four areas (Dolan, 2000). It is necessary in clinical trials to see if interventions are creating greater benefits than losses such as side effects; in individual patient care to improve clinical practice; in describing, monitoring and predicting population health; and in informing resource allocation decisions in healthcare.

A variety of measurements has been developed that tries to capture the utility of different health states, which usually involves having 'representative' individuals provide their preferences about different health states (Murray, 1996; Dolan, 2000; Dolan et al., 2005). The measurement in this exercise is not measuring whether an individual has a disease or its treatment, but measuring how much utility an individual gets from different states of mental and physical functioning in the spectrum between fully functioning and being dead. Based on what surveys or a panel of individuals states about these utility levels, using various statistical methods, valuations are produced for all health states. Once such measures are chosen, in all the four contexts mentioned above, the right and rational thing to do would be to pursue the action that maximizes the most health-welfare or health-utility.

However, what is morally troublesome with the general approach of utilitarianism is also not escaped by its specific application in the health domain. Health utilitarians seek to maximize health-utility through addressing the related physical and mental states in the population. If ten knee operations will create more utility than five hand operations, then the utilitarian will opt to do the knee operations. But then, things get a bit more complicated when the costs of operations are also included. Then the utilitarian will maximize the greatest utility per monetary unit. Meanwhile such a policy tolerates the impairments and preventable deaths of individuals whose resources needs are thought of as being cost-inefficient (Anand and Hanson, 1997; World Bank, 1997).[4] Similar to its hold on welfare economics, utilitarian reasoning in health economics and policy-making exhibits a number of defects.

Sen identifies utilarianism as having three components (Sen, 1999a, pp. 58–63). It is consequentialist in that it is focused on outcomes; it is welfarist in that what matters is welfare, or preference satisfaction; and it uses sum-ranking or aggregates utilities without a concern for distribution. The merits of utilitarianism are that it evaluates outcomes rather than steadfastly holding onto a position come what may.

A second virtue of this philosophy is that it focuses on human well-being rather than some abstract ideals or state of affairs. However, a purely welfarist view of health is inadequate for both its myopic focus only on 'health outcomes' while ignoring the moral relevance of the types of causes, persistence in populations, levels, full breadth of consequences and distribution patterns, as well as for disregarding the separateness of persons. In contrast, a capabilities approach could be focused on outcomes but include considerations across multiple dimensions, including causes and distribution.

Furthermore, as Nussbaum states with uncompromising clarity, aggregating across individuals, such as singularly aiming to maximize health-utility while sidelining the needs of the few – the minority – must be rejected because it is of supreme importance that we recognize 'a moral fact of paramount importance – that each person has only

one life to live . . .' (Nussbaum, 2006, p. 237). But there are many
utilitarians who simply find this unconvincing. They maintain that
resources are always finite, all individuals cannot be helped, and therefore, weighing lives is unavoidable and must be tackled head on. John
Broome even goes as far as to say that the Quality Adjusted Life Year
(QALY) measurement, the health utility measure popular in health
economics, should in fact be generalized to all human well-beings
(Broome, 2006, p. 261). Presumably, the idea would be to sum-rank
different amounts of 'well-being adjusted life years' in pursuing social
policy and justice.

There are many troubling aspects to each of the three characteristics
of utilitarianism that Sen identifies, and its application in relation to
health and longevity. Indeed, it is in the area of health that some of
the most convincing examples are found for why welfare or prefer-
ences/utility are not justifiable as the focal points of social justice.
Fundamentally, the difference lies in relying on individual's subjective
preferences about states of physical and mental functioning. Pain and
suffering from impairments are often the first and most compelling
aspects of a person that come to mind in reasoning about the moral
relevance of health. Yet, despite the external visibility of pain and suffering, people's valuation of their own physiological functioning is not
a good indicator of their claims for social support.

On the one hand, individuals suffering severe deprivation may consider it to be the normal way of living and thereby not express any
dissatisfaction. For example, pain thresholds are different for different
people but it seems wrong to make people bear more pain because they
can. On the other hand, individuals who are sufficiently functioning
may express intense dissatisfaction over minor impairments, be unduly
worried about non-visible impairments, or express frustration for not
possessing superior functionings. Or, once the necessary levels of subjective thresholds are made public, individuals can feign the intensity
to get care. While visible indications of pain and suffering, or physical
trauma may evidence impairments, the intensity of the pain and suffering a person exhibits is not a reliable indicator for the strength of
claims for social assistance. The 'happy-sick' or 'worried-well' both
point to the possible perverse results of relying wholly on subjective
desires or preferences.

Moreover, there is the additional problem when the preferences of
'expert panels' are used in health utility measurements. The question
of whose preferences about health states are to be included in the
health measurements within a given society is a difficult one. Should
they be of people while they are in states of impairment or people who

are not? Moreover, it seems fairly clear that it is even more problematic to use the preferences of an expert panel in constructing a health measurement to be applied across many countries. But that is exactly what is happening with the Disability Adjusted Life Year (DALY) measurement right now (Murray, 1994, 1996; World Health Organization, 2000).

So, in relying on utility measurements of health, there are problems of adaptive preferences, expensive preferences and even the imposition of preferences. Aside from the worry about adaptive preferences, Elizabeth Anderson offers the further criticisms that subjective utility should not serve as objects or metric of justice because of the publicity condition for social justice and because justice is about satisfying the needs of citizens 'to satisfy their objective interests as citizens' (Anderson, 2010, pp. 85–86). I think these points are important and worth mentioning but I do not pursue them here.

The persistence of welfarist thinking in health policy-making is driven largely by the pursuit of epidemiological and fiscal efficiency. For example, it is illuminating to see even the strongest advocates of the priority of liberty in social arrangements defer to the use of coercive measures during an epidemiological crisis. The threat of impairments or death from the transmission of pathogenic organisms is thought to be sufficient grounds to restrict fundamental liberties.[5] Such deference shows the extraordinary authoritative power of epidemiological science has to affect social arrangements. The goals of epidemiological efficiency suggest that the chosen course of action should be the one which will maximize the greatest number of disease cases averted, or the number of persons treated. During an infectious disease epidemic, pursuing epidemiological efficiency is often the motivation behind implementing coercive measures of social control on individuals who carry an infection or who are most likely to become infected, against a background of coercive measures applied widely across society.

But from the perspective of the capabilities approach, it is possible to argue that individuals who are carriers of a harmful infectious disease, or most vulnerable to it, exhibit acute failures of capabilities. These failures are in turn likely to have been preceded by endemic 'low intensity' capability failures. Drèze and Sen's analysis of endemic and acute malnutrition can easily be transposed onto the spread of infectious disease epidemics. An acute health crisis evidences the failure of social structures to ensure at least sufficient capabilities, particularly those relevant to biological functionings.

For example, the acute failures in the capabilities of poor girls and women to protect themselves from HIV is often merely the intensification of long-term endemic capability failures to achieving good reproductive and sexual health functionings. The spread of HIV/AIDS or other preventable infectious epidemics reflects capability failures. Indeed, the consistent neglect or sacrifice of the capabilities of those who are peripheral to the goal of cost-effectively maximizing total health utility of the population is often at the root of epidemiological crisis. Ironically as Jonathan Mann pointed out, epidemiological efficiency may be more achievable when societies ensure basic freedoms for all citizens than in following a course that restricts the liberties of those most vulnerable in the face of an epidemic (Mann et al., 1994; Mann, 1996, 1997).

The pervasiveness of utilitarian and welfarist reasoning in health policy is of course not limited to infectious diseases. It dominates the entire health policy-making process as well as the underlying science. In addressing chronic impairments, achieving epidemiological efficiency suggests that lowering the risk of the majority of individuals in the population slightly will prevent more cases of disease and, in the longer term, focus on the individuals who are most at risk (Rose, 1985). In statistical terms, lowering the mean-level exposure of the population will avert more cases of disease and be a more efficient expenditure of resources than trying to prevent disease in those with the highest exposure in the tails of the population. Such an analysis that pits the interests of the few against that of the many is familiar to philosophers as containing various defects but, in epidemiology and health policy, it is seen as offering clear guidance on the right course of social action. While improving the welfare of the majority of individuals, even by a little, may be a good thing to do, justice may require that we address the health capabilities of those individuals in the tails of the population especially if they are also socially disadvantaged in other ways. De-clustering disadvantage may outweigh the claims to the minor benefits that would be enjoyed by the majority (Wolff and De-Shalit, 2007).

The focus on the CH goes much further than welfarism in fully evaluating the moral relevance of the determinants, distribution, persistence and consequences of constraints on health capabilities and functionings. The CH argument presented here also clearly breaks down causes of health functionings as including personal features/ needs, conversion skills, exposures to external physical and social conditions. By focusing only on outcomes, utility maximization or welfarist theories exhibit a broad range of shortcomings in responding to health concerns. The value of freedom and respect for equal dignity of human beings compels evaluating multiple dimensions including the causes, distribution, consequences, possibilities of remedies and other aspects related to health. The foundational and Kantian liberal principle of 'each person as end' interpreted by Nussbaum as 'each person's capability' provides a strong basis for rejecting the singular focus on maximizing individual welfare or health-utility in addressing health concerns (Nussbaum, 2006, p. 216). In economic language, health justice demands an 'extra-welfarist' approach to health policy (Mooney, 2009).

Resource theories and health

An alternative to utility maximization is to focus on instrumental resources such as income, or on meeting basic needs. And in the domain of health, that has usually come to be seen as healthcare, broadly conceived as including clinical care, public health and health research. But the problem arises if such resource approaches only focus on goods, or maintain that justice requires giving only claims to resources. Reasoning that the moral concern for the health functionings of persons gives rise only to claims to healthcare resources, whether an 'essential package', or even more broadly defined healthcare goods and services, fails to take into account the diverse needs and endowments and varying conversion abilities of individuals in achieving any and all valuable health functioning. Claims only to a standard set of healthcare resources also exclude considering the possible non-healthcare material goods and social conditions necessary to maintaining physiological and agency functionings.

Healthcare is often valued for its restorative or ameliorative function. But for prevention, the 'upstream' requirements become much broader than even public health goods and services broadly defined. Goods and social conditions such as physical safety, access to income and freedom to access and share information are all crucial factors in determining the extent of vulnerability or risk to impairments and premature mortality (Commission on Social Determinants of Health, 2008; Marmot Review, 2010). The focus on healthcare alone does not fully appreciate the interaction of personal features, conversion skills, social conditions and the physical environment in the production of somatic and psychological functionings. Furthermore, aside from the diverse requirements just for the maintenance of functionings, the capabilities to deal with unforeseen threats over the life course that can cause impairments and premature mortality certainly require much more than clinical medical care and public health services.

Resource theories which do not even distribute healthcare specifically but expect income and wealth to satisfy the health needs of individuals over the life course especially evidence the inadequate ethical consideration of the determinants, consequences and distribution of human health functionings. For example, in his original theory Rawls excludes health concerns in identifying and distributing primary goods. Any additional material needs or difficulties in dealing with the social conditions in order to achieve, maintain, protect or restore health functionings are relegated to the personal sphere, or considered to be outside the scope of justice. Most importantly, individuals with severe and long-term impairments become second-class citizens as their 'extraordinary' needs are outside the scope of justice. Their interests are to be taken care of by guardians. The financial costs and non-financial resources such as time and energy of others needed to provide care are invisible from the calculation of primary goods. In the extreme, when personal resources and/or public beneficence are not enough to achieve sufficient health functionings, the constraints consequently restrict, if not fully extinguish, the practical possibility of an individual to pursue their own ends.[6] That is to say, prudential contractors in a hypothetical contract would want to put limits on the amount of resources that any single person could claim, and when this amount runs out, the individual would become dependent on charity of fellow citizens (Pogge, 1989, 1995; Kittay, 1997; Pogge, 2004; Nussbaum, 2006; Terzi, 2010).

Resource theory advocates either have a blind spot to this significant consequence or are willing to accept this sort of inequality in substantive freedom caused by health constraints. They highlight the possible role of individual volitional choices and preferences in creating extra health needs and, therefore, their justifiable exclusion from legitimate claims for social support. For example, health needs that are caused directly from participating in dangerous sports or smoking would not have to be met as a matter of justice because the individuals knowingly chose to place themselves in that position of risk (Fleurbaey, 2008; Segall, 2009). Such a focus on personal accountability may alleviate some guilt for resourcists, but it does not fully manage to make up for the injustice in the price paid by the remaining individuals who may be the most vulnerable of all members of society; individuals who did nothing to expose themselves to harm but whose health-related costs exceed the standard set of entitlements. The situation is not only tragic because such individuals cannot have their resource needs satisfied, it is also insulting to the individuals to be told that justice does not require providing such resources.

This disregard or inadequate consideration of the needs of individuals outside of the 'standard conception' violates the fundamental principle of showing equal concern to all members of society. Moreover, the emphasis on choice versus luck places resourcists in the position of having to assume the causation of the health impairment is clear and established; it either has to be a result of choices or brute luck. Otherwise, how would one determine whether the person is responsible for their own extra health needs? (Cohen, 1989; Roemer, 1993; Cohen, 1997; Fleurbaey, 2008).[7] What these resourcists also miss is that every human being at one time or another over the life course will experience severe impairments that will make them dependent on others. And it is quite certain that human societies will continue to experience major health crises in the immediate future. Human beings are and will continue to be vulnerable and interdependent human beings. A standard set of primary goods or healthcare resources does not adequately account for the different needs and vulnerabilities of human beings over the life course or provide security against changing threats to the embodied functionings of the human species (Wolff and De-Shalit, 2007, pp. 63–73). Rather than focus on the means, why not focus on ensuring their capabilities, what individuals can be and do over the life course?

In that process of abstracting away from the personal features, choices or preferences that individuals may make or have in order to reflect on the just distribution of resources, resourcists do not seem to exhibit a thorough understanding of the causes, consequences and distribution of mortality and impairments among human beings. For example, in responding to Rawls, Ronald Dworkin specifically identifies differences in physical and mental abilities as constituting morally relevant inequalities in personal resources under one's command. Dworkin then goes on to argue that the sufficient social response to addressing physical and mental impairments should take the form of providing additional compensation to those who had no control over the cause of those impairments (Dworkin, 1993, 2000).

Although Dworkin rightly recognizes the moral relevance of health impairments, his analysis is too simplistic for idealizing health functionings as being caused either by innate features or volitional choices. And he seems to see no problem with reasoning that the effects of either a temporary or permanent impairment on a person's life can be justly addressed through individual, monetary compensation. One objection to monetary compensation is that impairments can impinge on equal dignity, and may not be just about monetary compensation for loss of social advantage. It may be that social conditions need to change. A second concern is that disability results in both earnings handicap (inadequate or low income) and conversion handicap (disadvantage converting earnings into good living) (Sen, 2004b, pp. 258–260; Kuklys, 2005; Sen, 2009). Disabled individuals may require both additional income as well as assistance with converting resources into pursuing their plans of life.

Viewed from the perspective of capabilities, resource theories are inadequate with respect to what they include and exclude in their standard conception of persons, what they consider morally relevant features of persons. Resource theories are also inadequate for looking at intermediary resource holdings to assess how well the lives of people are going. Indeed, Rawls and resourcists after him do recognize human diversity. But such diversity is seen in the varying conceptions of the good, and the differing effects on a person's life course caused by the (supposedly) random and unequal distribution of natural goods (talents, skills, intelligence, health), volitional choices and random events of bad luck.

The CA does not deny the moral significance of the human capacity for moral reasoning in conceiving the good, the differences in innate qualities, the role of volitional choices, or even bad luck. However, the CA recognizes more fully the moral relevance of how every human being is, as G. A. Cohen states, differently 'constructed and situated' (Cohen, 1989). The lack of sufficient recognition and consideration of the diversity of human beings in their needs and abilities to convert their own endowments and external social and physical conditions into life's beings and doings results in significant challenges for resource theories.

Daniels' health justice

But it seems, according to what Norman Daniels has been writing most recently, his version of the Rawlsian theory addresses many of the weakness of resource approaches and is virtually the same as the capabilities approach (Daniels, 2010). Daniels' assertion that there are very few meaningful differences between his extension of the best available resource theory and the capabilities approach compels closer examination. It is also interesting that it is through accommodating for health issues that the best resource theory, Rawls' theory, and the capabilities approach are seen to come together. At the core, Daniels argues that fair equality of opportunity which Rawls tries to provide through primary goods, and which is further corrected for health impairments by Daniels, is the same space as capabilities equity that Sen and Nussbaum advance (Daniels, 2008, pp. 64–71, 2010, p. 134).

I would argue that important differences remain between resource and capabilities theories, and that Daniels' argument has still got some difficulties even after his revisions. And it should be unsurprising that I would argue that the CH argument can still do better in addressing health concerns. Yet, I do think it is worth at least briefly addressing Daniels' theory. This discussion presupposes the reader has some familiarity with Rawls' theory of justice.

Daniels initially engages with Rawls' theory from recognizing that individuals with equal primary goods would not be equally well-off from the perspective of justice if they had different health-care needs (Daniels, 1985, p. 43). Two individuals with the same income but with different healthcare needs could have dramatically different quality of life. This was a consequence of Rawls' idealizing assumption that all individuals in his society would be healthy from birth to death. Daniels wanted to take away this assumption, but access to healthcare which could make people with different healthcare needs more equal could not simply be added to the list. Kenneth Arrow had pointed out a decade earlier this same point and that putting healthcare on the list would create two problems (Arrow, 1973). Given Rawls required that socio-economic inequalities must work to the advantage of the worst-off, individuals with severe health resource needs could bankrupt the society. And, putting healthcare on the list and allowing a trade-off between it and income and wealth would create the problem of having to compare utilities of individuals rather than look just at their holdings of primary goods.

So Daniels' move was to focus instead on one of the existing primary goods on the list, the fair equality of opportunity (Daniels, 1985, p. 45). He broadened Rawls' fair equality of opportunity to achieve jobs and offices into a fair equality of opportunity to pursue a normal opportunity range (NOR) of life plans for a society. As a person's health impacts their fair equality of opportunity, and there is a causal link between healthcare and health, Daniels argued that individuals should have entitlements to healthcare. Because society has an obligation to provide the resource of equality of opportunity, society will guarantee access to healthcare. Consequently, healthcare institutions should be understood as one of the basic institutions of society that function to ensure equality of opportunity of citizens to pursue life plans. And, importantly, healthcare is to be distributed according to its impact on the fair equality of opportunity of citizens to pursue the NOR within a society.

Daniels' initial argument became well known within the field of bioethics and health policy discussions in the United States. And his argument also received a boost when Rawls noted that he generally supported Daniels' approach to addressing health needs (Rawls, 1993, p. 184; Rawls and Kelly, 2001, p. 171). Nevertheless, Daniels himself has recently identified its shortcomings (Daniels, 2007). He readily identifies the theory's lack of practical guidance in making resource allocation decisions simply based on the effects of health impairments on equality of opportunity. He writes that reasonable people disagree on the different principles to use in deciding how to allocate healthcare resources. And second, he admits to the egregiously generous causal connection made between healthcare and health that ignores the more significant social determinants of health as well as the lack of a broader 'population health' perspective. He made two revisions to his theory to address the shortcomings. It now includes a list of principles of fairness to aid the decision-making process of allocating healthcare resources. And he incorporates social determinants of health research, and a population health perspective. He argues that serendipitously it turns out that Rawls' theory of justice captures key social determinants of health meaning that a Rawlsian society would justly distribute social determinants of health (Daniels et al., 1999; Daniels, 2008).

Daniels' reasoning proceeds in the following way. He identifies a conception of health, what objective 'health needs' there are related to health, why health is important to human beings and then, what social obligations there are to ensure people achieve good health. He conceives health as species typical functioning based on Boorse's arguments. Then he identifies six 'health needs' which include (1) adequate nutrition, (2) safe living and working conditions, (3) exercise and rest, (4) medical services, (5) non-medical personal and social services, and (6) an appropriate distribution of social determinants of health (Daniels, 2008, pp. 42–43).

Meeting these needs is necessary in order to protect normal functioning, which in turn protects access to the fair share of the range of life prospects. Rational individuals, such as those behind Rawls' veil of ignorance, will want to maintain their normal functionings to pursue as well as revise their life plans, and the equality of opportunity to pursue the normal range of life plans. Therefore, rational individuals will make sure that social institutions will satisfy the six objective 'health needs' of citizens.

Daniels' theory versus the CH

From the perspective of an advocate of the capabilities approach, I do believe that Daniels has indeed presented a compelling resource theory account of health justice. He presents a non-subjective account of health-related claims. And he has rightly recognized that health is determined by more than healthcare as he now includes the broader social determinants of health. But we should note that this resulted from a chance encounter with social epidemiologists rather than being driven by a demand internal to his theory to be vigilant for such knowledge of the social bases of health (Daniels, 2008, p. 4). In any case, there is also an overlap between his concern for the fair opportunity for individuals to pursue life plans and the focus of the capabilities approach on ensuring individuals have opportunity through being practically able to pursue their life plans, their beings and doings. But there are a number of weaknesses in Daniels' argument. I shall focus on his 'natural' baseline of health, the list of health-needs and the incorporation of social determinants of health,

Following Rawls, Daniels works with two sources of inequalities in the lives of individuals. Inequalities that come from the natural lottery and those from the social lottery. The natural lottery determines the quality and breadth of psychological and somatic talents and skills which one is endowed with at birth. It also affects motivational traits, attitudes and preferences to some extent.[8] The social lottery encompasses early-life conditions determined by family, caste/class and so forth. Such early life environments are also thought to affect psychological traits such as preferences and motivational traits. Rawls took the natural lottery as a neutral baseline, a 'natural good', and aimed to correct the arbitrary disadvantages that arise from the social malformations of the talents and skills a person is 'naturally' born with. In recognizing that those with naturally lesser talents and skills would be at the bottom of the social hierarchy, even after the arbitrary social influences had been corrected, he aims to ensure that they are as advantaged as much as possible. All socio-economic inequalities are to work to the advantage of the worst-off.

Daniels builds on Rawls' analysis of the arbitrary inequalities created by the natural and social lottery by making an analogy between pathology and the social lotteries. Just as there is an ethical requirement to counter the disadvantages experienced by individuals from their early social environment or to balance out the advantages some individuals get from their social environment, Daniels argues that there is a requirement to mitigate the disadvantages produced by pathology (Daniels, 2008, p. 58). While he does not use the term 'pathological lottery', it may be apt to describe his analysis.

Moreover, Daniels implies that given the recent research on social determinants of health, the analogy between pathology and the social lottery becomes even closer. Pathology in an individual can arise from the social environment, 'including class, gender, race and ethnic inequalities in various goods' and, therefore, any disadvantages that follow are not deserved and should be mitigated from affecting a person's life prospects (Daniels, 2008, p. 58).

Daniels' aim is to restore people to where their health would be had there been no impairments caused by lack of health-needs and the negative social influences. But it is the notion of comparing individuals to a neutral, natural baseline that is the problem. The distribution of health functionings in a population, such as longevity, is inherently determined by social processes. For human beings, unlike for fruit-flies or zebras, longevity and physiological functioning are socially influenced and therefore cannot be morally neutral. It is like taking the life expectancy of different societies as natural, or morally neutral, even though we know that the different life expectancies are not due to biology but because of the social structures and processes affecting that society. People are also born with impairments built into them caused by social factors affecting previous generations. Though an individual has no control over her initial natural endowments, the social environment did influence them. A person's natural endowments are the product of the endowments of their parents. And how and when the parents procreated is profoundly affected by social conditions (Posner, 1992, Bauman, 2003). Daniels, however, holds onto a natural baseline as being neutral, and then intends to regulate the social determinants of health during the individual's lifetime to keep her within the natural or neutral distribution. This is implausible. Both the inequalities from the natural and social lotteries have to be recognized and addressed in reasoning about the opportunities individuals have in pursuing their life plans.

A second aspect that is incongruent in Daniels' argument is his list of health-needs. His revised list of needs is the same as his previous list of healthcare needs broadly construed plus 'appropriate distribution of social determinants of health'. It is unclear how this list of health-needs has been constructed. There is no epidemiological theory or even a salutogenic theory that would explain the components of the list. Moreover, adding social determinants at the end of the list actually repeats some of the items on the list. It perhaps expresses Daniels' understanding of social determinants as psychosocial determinants of health versus what Sen identifies as broad social arrangements. For example, including adequate nutrition and safe working environment as needs along with social determinants of health as a need does not fully appreciate the 'general theory' of social determinants of health research.

Additionally, social determinants of health research is actually research on the social determinants of impairments and mortality, not of health and longevity. Social determinants of health are usually 'bads' – income inequality, low control, low agency, discrimination and so forth. But Daniels seems to have understood social determinants as good things and has paired them up with Rawls' primary goods. Or, we have to assume that he has simply transformed the causes of disease and mortality into their positive correlates without sufficient explanation of how that is done. That would be something that even epidemiologists would be nervous about doing; a cause of disease does not automatically tell us what is to be done to prevent or mitigate it. Also, by selectively picking from the variety of proposed determinants, Daniels skips over discussing the important distinction in the causal pathways between social determinants of health of a group versus an individual. Without an identifiable link between the health properties of a group and an individual, Daniels seems to be making arguments for group justice rather than arguing for a theory where individuals are primary moral agents. He argues that a population has been treated badly if its overall health is worse than it could have been under another policy. How a 'population perspective' and a Rawlsian system can go together is not fully defended, especially as Rawls was motivated to counter utilitarian reasoning. No individual can make a direct claim with regard to social determinants affecting their health as the social pathways to impairments are identified in aggregate statistics, not in the case of particular individuals. So, under this system, health inequalities caused by social determinants become unjust only at the population level, not at the individual level.

One important thing that resourcists like Daniels and capabilities theorists alike must recognize is that experiences of social inequality such as from income differences or through discrimination based on race, gender or sexuality cannot be understood as simply an absence of a resource or primary good. When conceiving of individuals as pursuing mutual advantage, discrimination looks like the denial of equal access or opportunity to the pursuit of life plans. Yet, in the context of health functionings, discrimination is not just the absence of primary goods such as social basis of self-respect, or lack of equality of opportunity. Perennial stress and anxiety from discrimination gets converted through psycho-biological pathways into impairments and early death. The lack of primary goods does not mean just the lack of instrumental means but also that it is a source of direct harm. The capability space, by being grounded in dignity, and focused on ensuring a sufficient level of opportunity and activity is not only instrumentally and intrinsically valuable, it can also be protective. Ensuring a sufficient level of capabilities means that the human animal's neediness, sociability and ability to reason are not only allowed to function but that such functioning is protected and nurtured because it is necessary for its survival.

Luck egalitarianism

Over the last thirty years a group of academic philosophers have developed the view that the essence of egalitarianism – what follows from the equal moral worth of persons – lies in neutralizing the effects of bad luck on a person's life prospects; that a society or government showing equal concern and respect means mitigating the disadvantages caused by factors over which an individual has no control. To have any meaning, such a view also requires holding people responsible for the consequences of what they can control or could have controlled including the risks taken. But holding such a view has some unpalatable consequences in the domain of healthcare. Individuals who are ill because of their imprudent choices have to be abandoned. That is, according to egalitarian justice, it is right to provide healthcare to those who need it because they are naturally or socially unlucky, but those individuals who are ill and indeed at risk of death because of their own negligence do not have any claims on society for assistance. In fact, imprudent individuals can be seen as avoidably burdening the health system, taking away resources from unlucky individuals, and are unfair to those who at least do try making prudent decisions.

Shlomi Segall is attempting to save luck egalitarianism from its inhumane ultimate conclusions in the domain of healthcare as well as from being rejected more broadly as an approach to social justice (Segall, 2009). The meanness of abandoning the negligent victim was highlighted by Elizabeth Anderson as one of several weaknesses of luck egalitarian justice in a devastating and now seminal essay titled, 'What is the Point of Equality?' (Anderson, 1999). Segall endeavours to escape the charge of meanness as well as develop a luck egalitarian argument for universal and unconditional healthcare, working through how luck egalitarianism would address social determinants of health and the health gradient, human enhancement technology, devolution of healthcare services and global health inequalities.

Segall's position is that abandoning the imprudent is the right logical conclusion, but that more fundamental or prior moral social commitments such as that of meeting basic needs would intercede to provide care to the imprudent patient. He defends this resolution to the dilemma by arguing that luck egalitarianism is only a part of morality, and that we use various other values to design and judge social institutions aside from fairness. Moreover, this notion of a longstanding or foundational ethical commitment to meeting basic needs includes medical care needs, and makes healthcare something that cannot be withheld from anyone. This inability to deny anyone basic needs then leads to providing universal healthcare to all residents within national borders. Nevertheless, where scarce resources force a choice between one who was prudent but unlucky and one who was imprudent, Segall suggests a lottery slightly weighted in favour of the innocent party. Providing some chance of getting healthcare is said to provide escape from the meanness objection. But it is ironic that applying a theory that seeks to neutralize bad luck nevertheless leads Segall to rely on a luck mechanism to determine life or death decisions.

I disagree with Segall about the extent to which luck egalitarianism constitutes a substantive theory of justice and, therefore, how satisfactorily it illuminates what to do about the issues he focuses on or other troubling health issues facing us. Segall is aware of the work of Sen and Nussbaum, and uses their ideas and quotes at important points in his arguments. But he misleadingly presents health justice debates as largely shaped by and occurring between Rawlsians and luck egalitarians. It is not insignificant that Sen used physical disability as the illustrative example to highlight what is wrong with Rawls' theory and broader egalitarian thought in his 1979 Tanner lecture before advocating for basic capability equality. And Nussbaum has written extensively on moral luck, which informs her arguments for entitlements to central human capabilities such as to life and bodily health. These are the same arguments that intercede here to save the imprudent patient. The fact Segall draws on Nussbaum's entitlements to basic capabilities or something like basic needs in order to save his theory, I would argue, does more to advance the capabilities approach than luck egalitarianism as a viable approach to health justice.

Conclusion

The aim of the chapter was to compare and contrast the argument for the CH with alternative ethical approaches. Such a process is an ongoing and necessary part of the dialectical reasoning required for reasoning about the basic principles of social justice. As the discussion shows, I argue that the CH does a better job of theorizing and realizing health justice than do other ethical approaches and general theories. But ethical reasoning, like science, is dependent on public scrutiny. In both domains, knowledge is expanded through the coherence and acceptance of the analyses and arguments, which depends on their being able to withstand public scrutiny. So I expect these arguments will need to be modified or supplemented; it is an ongoing process. I would readily acknowledge one weakness of the CH argument, and CA more generally. Groups, whether small or national populations, present a challenge to the CA that puts individuals as the objects of ultimate moral concern. That is the subject of the next chapter.

6

Groups and Capabilities

In this chapter, I present some of the issues related to groups that arise in trying to extend the CA into the domain of health. Indeed, some of these issues will arise in any liberal theory of justice that takes the individual as the primary moral agent, and seeks to integrate research on the social determinants of health and align itself with a population health perspective. At the same time, there are murmurings in the circles of capabilities theorists about group capabilities also being a target of ethical concern, a metric of justice, just like the capabilities of individuals (Gore, 1997; Majumdar and Subramanian, 2001; Sen, 2002b; Stewart and Deneulin, 2002; Robeyns, 2005a; Stewart, 2005).

The first discussion about analysis of health issues at the population level and the second discussion about group capabilities obviously intersect. However, because of the strong causal relationship I am making between social institutions and processes and impairment and mortality, how we reason about groups and health capabilities has far-reaching consequences for the capabilities approach. To be clearer, the issue is not 'just' about whether a group can have claims to certain artistic culture or language that is created through social interaction. It is more fundamental in that the social values and social processes of a group are correlated with the causation and distribution of premature mortality and impairments. Put simply, does a group have a claim to produce, protect, sustain and promote 'population health'?

Let me begin with the argument of Paula Braveman and Sofia Gruskin. In seeking to improve and clarify Margaret Whitehead's three health equity principles, they advance the definition of equity in health as 'the absence of systematic disparities in health (or in the major social determinants of health) between social groups who have different levels of underlying social advantage/disadvantage – that is, different positions in a social hierarchy' (Braveman and Gruskin, 2003, p. 254). They continue by stating: 'Inequities in health systematically put groups of people who are already socially disadvantaged (for example, by virtue of being poor, female and/or members of a disenfranchised racial, ethnic or religious group) at further disadvantage with respect to their health . . .' It should be fairly clear that Braveman and Gruskin are defining health equity only in terms of group inequalities. They emphasize the inequity in the correlation of (a) health outcomes and the social determinants of health with (b) social groups with different social advantage. What do they have to say about inter-individual health inequalities? Even Brian Barry, whom I quoted in the Introduction, seems to be focused on the justice and health of groups. He writes: 'Wherever we find groups with a 'structural characteristic' that experiences differences in their health, it is a *prima facie* unjust distribution' (Barry, 2005, p. 73). Perhaps this is understandable as most of the social epidemiology and health equity literature is about the differences in health outcomes between social groups, usually socio-economic groups. This kind of analysis gives rise to thinking of injustice between groups. Or, put in another way, given the analysis of social determinants of health and social inequalities in health happens at the group level, what ethical claims do individuals have regarding the social determinants of health?

If we are right to integrate the causes, persistence, distribution, levels, consequences and possible remedies of impairments and mortality systematically within a general theory of justice, considering the justice of health differences only at the social group level would mean that we would need a theory of justice that gives groups ethical status. It is inconsistent to talk about inequity or injustice between groups without linking it to individuals within a theory of justice that takes individuals as the ultimate units of moral concern. So how does the empirical analysis of social inequalities in health in order to identify social determinants of health, and Braveman and Gruskin's idea that group health differences are a matter of equity and justice align with the capabilities approach? An approach, which I must emphasize, whose advocates are usually vehement about asserting individual human beings as the ultimate or basic units of moral concern. Is there something about what is visible or happening at the *population health* level that should motivate us to identify group entitlements to health capabilities?

Ethical individualism

Many sociologists, social epidemiologists and public health practitioners may find this worry and anxiety over the moral status of groups to be perplexing, if not amusing. Surely, in this day and age, it would be surprising to find people denying that society consists of more than the sum of individuals; that society can be understood from looking at individuals. While it may be true that there is much knowledge still to be learned or publicly disseminated about the social aspects of individual health and individual well-being more generally, the moral worry here is about the ethical status, not the sociological aspects of groups. Remember that the motivating concerns behind the CA were to counter the promotion of aggregate wealth of nations (i.e. groups) without consideration of distribution across individuals, and to address the persistent inequalities in well-being across individuals. Concerns for individual well-being motivate the starting point that the individual human being should be the primary agent of moral concern, and of justice.

Such an approach is distinct from other approaches that start with a conception of community in reasoning about social justice or with the nation-state when thinking about global justice (Walzer, 1983; Kymlicka, 1989; Taylor, 1992; Sandel, 1996; Rawls, 1999). Furthermore, even though many liberal theories purport to begin with the individual as the moral agent, they implicitly assume insiders and outsiders of a community. Thus, the existence of outsiders means they start with an insider group prior to reasoning about justice and individual moral agents (Sen, 2005; Nussbaum, 2006). The CA unequivocally begins with the individual. And as discussed in Part II, it also differentiates itself from other liberal theories that focus on distributing resources to individuals or increasing their welfare. The CA strives to avoid the inequalities across individuals that result from the aggregate maximization analysis used by utilitarians. It also strives to avoid the inequalities that arise under resource theories when individual needs for goods or social conditions fall outside the standard set of entitlements. That is, in resource theories extra-standard needs due to variations in natural endowments and needs or conversion skills are seen to fall outside the scope of what society is obligated to provide.

In contrast, because the CA is exclusively focused on individual capabilities, or guaranteeing a minimum set of CHCs, the CA appears to avoid aggregate analysis within or across individuals. It does not presuppose the aim of maximizing capabilities or that there will be a need to put caps on per-person resource expenditures to pre-empt drain on social resources. Nevertheless, the CA almost certainly cannot avoid aggregating capabilities within and across individuals as it is a practical issue central to implementation at the level of social policy.

Considering the entitlements to individual capabilities and difficulties about how to aggregate individual capabilities in order to implement policy makes visible something at the group level not visible when thinking about individuals. When we start thinking about aggregating individual capabilities, there is conceptual difficulty because the capabilities approach exhibits forms of ontological or explanatory individualism. The singular concern for individual capabilities makes it seem as though the only things of moral relevance are individuals, and that everything can be explained in terms of individuals. Manabi Majumdar and S. Subramanian resist this kind of capabilities approach. In pursuing the measurement of group differences in capability failures they write: '. . . personal destinies, and indeed personal identities, are frequently bound up so intimately in group affiliations that the resulting patterns of social stratification which emerge are quite entirely lost to social analysis when a thoroughgoing "individualistic" approach to inequality assessment is adopted' (Majumdar and Subramanian, 2001, p. 105). But clearly, the capabilities approach is not wholly individualistic. Many of the capabilities that Nussbaum advocates are based on the sociability of human beings and reflect interdependence. And Sen as well as others discuss various capabilities that are related to social interactions and those that are formed through social interaction. But even if the CA recognizes that individuals belong to groups, does it represent groups as being understandable by looking at individuals? Does the CA express a kind of view that group characteristics are only made up of the additive characteristics of individuals? If the CA does not deny holism, then are CA advocates simply being more vocal about individuals' capabilities, while remaining silent about the possible emergent properties of groups and their claims to capabilities?

Group capabilities initially seem to be an abhorrent concept to anyone espousing the CA; for a number of very good reasons. For example, the CA vehemently rejects the utilitarian aggregation of the welfare of individuals as if it were the welfare of a 'super-person'; it violates the principle of treating each person separately and each as their own end. Yet, certain kinds of health phenomena and their underlying sociological processes cannot be disaggregated to the actions of individual agents. Recalling Geoffrey Rose, he argued for recognizing the important difference in addressing the cause of impairments in individuals versus the causes of the incidence rate of the impairment in the population (Rose, 1985). There are two levels of analysis in public health, one at the individual level, and one at the population level (Kelly et al., 2010). Most people who work in social epidemiology or health sociology are very familiar and comfortable with this concept. But 'population health' presents interesting challenges for any ethical approach which recognizes the individual as the primary agent of justice.

However, as it is recognizable that some populations and sub-populations are healthy, while others are less so, there appears to be a need to integrate such a population health notion into the CA through the idea of a group capability and group CH (Wilkinson, 1996; Mooney, 2005; Wilkinson and Pickett, 2009). Or, putting it differently, improving the CH of individuals will not improve the health of the population; the problem of the persistence of deprivations through generations continues as the causal determinants of the deprivations can still be functioning in the background as the capability of each individual is protected. It is the diversity in these background social conditions that, for example, produce differing levels of motor vehicle accidents or homicides in different societies, but remain constant across years in each society. So the concern for the persistence of impairments and mortality through generations may require acting at the population level, with only a rough idea, rather than exact idea, of which individuals might benefit.

In contrast to the research in social epidemiology, the CA recognizes group or social phenomena only through their influence on individual capabilities and the expression of certain capabilities. That is, social phenomena enter capabilities analysis through the social basis of the causal components of individual capabilities. And sociability of the human animal is expressed in the specific content of capabilities such as some of Nussbaum's CHCs. Societies or groups are never considered as entities with independent ethical status alongside individuals. Indeed, CA theorists may consider it useful to describe the capabilities of members of a particular group. A group of individuals can be said to exhibit a certain kind of capability or be constrained in a particular way. The Senian capability device, for example, can be applied to any sort of capability and does not restrict the holders of the capability to individuals. The idea of a group capability presents a problem only in the normative realm when ascribing ethical status and entitlements to capabilities.

Foremost among the worries is the possibility of a conflict between group and individual capabilities. That is to say, group capabilities can be advanced at the cost of the capabilities of individuals within the group. And primary attention to group capabilities may not give sufficient attention to inequalities in capabilities of individuals within the group. The violence that can be perpetrated and justified by utilitarians in the name of maximizing aggregate welfare could also happen in the name of improving group capabilities. In order to avoid this, there is a burden to show how doing group level analysis and reducing group inequities such as in health outcomes benefits individuals within groups, and that the benefits are distributed fairly across individuals.

Health and collective action problems

In contrast to the social contract tradition which conceives of individuals as being purely self interested and seeking mutual advantage, the CA sees social cooperation as being made possible through individuals conceiving their good as having shared ends. The incorporation of the pursuit of the good by others into one's own conception of the good is what defines interdependence, fellowship and sociability of human beings. However, the conception of individuals as self-interested actors has been longstanding, compelling and pervasive. And, there are many types of problems such a conception of persons create for social cooperation.

Examination of the implications of a self-interested individual can be seen in political philosophy as well as the sub-field of economics which considers problems of collective action and cooperative conflicts. Until fairly recently, the social or collective action aspect of human health functionings has been largely under-explored due to the general perception that health is an individual level phenomenon. It must be recalled that the most prominent model of health causation focuses on individual-level factors of genetic endowment, exposure to proximate hazardous materials and behaviours. Individuals and their health are seen in a vacuum, devoid of any social context. This is not to say that health and social cooperation problems have not been considered at all.

The influence of economics in the practice of public health has motivated the framing of some health issues as collective action problems, public goods and externalities. For example, in the study of population growth, fertility decisions are often framed as being made by self-interested individuals causing burdens on aggregate welfare, individuals producing negative externalities. Or healthcare expenditures are analysed in reference to 'moral-hazards' or self-interested individuals unfairly or deceptively taking advantage of group resources. In these types of situations, instead of an individual's good being seen as being constituted partly by another achieving their conception of the good, certain self-interested individuals are seen to be violating the principle of mutual advantage that underpins social cooperation between individuals.

The collective action or group-level problems in the health sphere have become more pronounced recently in light of at least two phenomena. First, the rise of new and resurgent infectious diseases has made it abundantly clear that the mortality of human beings is a function of the interactions between individuals within and across national borders. In its clearest example, the transmission of infection from one individual to another is a social phenomenon. But it is also clear that the social environment in which individuals are situated also determines their biological vulnerability to infectious diseases as well as their ability to mitigate their vulnerability. The second collective action aspect of health is reflected in the social epidemiological research that identifies social processes as determinants of health functionings. That is, social processes not only determine the material exposure to harmful access to necessary goods affecting health functionings; social interactions and institutions influence individual agency, autonomy, dignity and other psychological experiences which then affect the biological pathways of a person's health over the life course. Some of this research was discussed in Chapter 2.

Based on aggregate analysis, it is possible to identify the social cause of the incidence rate of impairments in a population. But it may be impossible to connect a social determinant to a particular impairment in a particular individual. As a result, the scope of ethical claims at the individual level would be limited, as it would only be possible to definitely identify the proximate biological, material causes along with behavioural causes of the impairment. A theory of causation plays an important role here. Without a theory of causation connecting social determinants to the impairment or death of a specific individual, it would be difficult to assert that individual's CH has been violated. But an individual could make a positive claim for certain social conditions because they are likely to benefit her as she belongs to a group that would probably benefit. This is partly the idea behind Sen's meta-right, a right to social policies that aim to realize the content of a right. Or, the individual could also argue that the lack of social conditions could have probably caused her impairments, given that she is a member of a group that has suffered under such social conditions.

Reasoning such as this, then, begins the slippery slope of identifying the claims of unspecified individuals belonging to various groups. But does doing something in the interests of unspecified individuals belonging to a certain group constitute giving ethical status to a group? Utilitarians would see no problem here, as influencing the social determinants would increase the aggregate welfare of the group, even if benefits could not be traced to particular individuals. But normative individualists have a significant problem because there is no clear causal pathway between the structure and the individual.

An economist might immediately frame this as a public goods issue. A public good is a good that no single individual can consume exclusively, and the amount of the good does not decrease from being consumed. For example, draining a malaria-infested swamp next to a community of individuals is considered providing a public good. Draining the swamp in order to benefit one individual could not exclude its benefits to others. And the benefit to one individual does not decrease the amount of the good. Seen from the perspective of the CA, providing such a public good protects the health capabilities and functionings or CH of individuals living next to the drained swamp. Such an effort is considered to be focused on individual capabilities because it is addressing the material, social bases of each person's health capability. We know that a mosquito bite is probably part of the causal chain that leads to an individual's being impaired. Thus, based on the knowledge of the causal pathway, the public good is provided in order to support the capabilities of individuals living within the community.

However, when the cause of the impairment is social conditions which induce psychological experiences such as humiliation or stress, which then lead to health impairments, it is hard to separate out the public good from the intrinsic features of the population. The malarial swamp as a physical feature and the social conditions of inequality are not equivalent in a way that both can be addressed through the public goods framework. Material conditions may be more amenable to be assessed as public goods, while certain psychosocial processes need to be recognized as group features. Take another example: protecting the

CH of individuals could be the basis of programmes to help individuals quit smoking, a widely recognized cause of lung cancer.

However, helping one individual at a time to stop smoking, according to the each person's capability as an end principle, would not necessarily stop new individuals from beginning to smoke. The causes which initiate individuals into smoking continue to function in the surrounding social environment. The same applies to other behaviours such as poor nutrition, or excessive drinking. In order to intervene at the level of supra-individual influences on individual behaviour, such as culture, social norms, neighbourhood effects and so forth, we would have to acknowledge that individuals are not fully autonomous but partly or significantly formed by social practices. What ethical status do these supra-individual influences, which cannot be ascribed to any individual agent, but yet significantly influence individual capabilities, have in the CA? It is insufficient to think of social conditions or influences on individual capabilities as simply being the combined actions of other individuals.

In fact, recognizing the causal factors of constraints on individual health capability absolutely requires recognizing the characteristics of social groups or populations. When comparing different possible causal factors of a chronic impairment among individuals within a population, individual genetic differences are often statistically significant factors of causation. In the CA, such genetic bases of a health constraint would be the basis for providing social support. Interestingly, however, when comparing two significantly different populations with different prevalence levels of the same chronic impairment, individual genetic differences become less important as causal factors than differences in population characteristics.

For example, individual genetic differences may be identified as significant causes or risk-factors for the high prevalence of heart disease in residents of Finland. But when comparing the causes of heart disease in the populations of Finland versus Japan, the average intake of fat and high cholesterol levels become significant factors. Because fat intake is high for most individuals in Finland, it does not appear as a statistically significant causal factor within the Finnish population. Thus, the only real differences between those with and without high cholesterol and heart disease within Finland are individual genetic differences. The upshot of this is that the methodology of identifying causal factors of health functionings in individuals can involve comparing groups, and not necessarily only individuals.

Once population-level differences are understood to be causal factors in the prevalence of impairments and mortality, the most effective way of reducing such ill-health is to change the mean-level of exposure of the population level; it requires shifting the entire population, changing social norms regarding the risk factors. Changing the mean level of exposure of the entire group would mean an intervention to change a feature affecting the aggregate capabilities of the group for the long term, even generations. Thus, despite specific individuals benefiting in differing amounts from an intervention or policy at a particular time, the primary beneficiary is actually the group. By changing the group feature, the collective health capability is improved and kept above a threshold even as people pass through it by birth and death. So now, draining the swamp looks different from this perspective. It cannot be simply thought that the CH of a large group of individuals is improved because of the features of a public good and its efficiency. Rather, the policy also improves the collective CH of the community in that location, irrespective of which individual is there currently or will pass through in the future. Changing social conditions, whether they are material conditions or social processes, which are aimed to outlast specific individuals, are really efforts at changing the features of groups, and thus, group capabilities.

Addressing the cause of any impairment in an individual across the range of causal components is distinct from addressing the incidence rate of the impairment in the population. The reach of the CH causal model in explaining how social determinants that have influence through psychobiological pathways and their varied effects across socio-economic groups are yet to be explored. It seems easy to fall into thinking of a social group as a 'super-person' and explore social policies that can improve the super-person's 'population health' or capability. Difficult ethical questions follow from giving a population its own ethical status, and from making decisions using aggregate analysis. But it is hard to deny that individual health and population health are two distinct, inter-related phenomena.

I have no easy answer here aside from an intuitive scepticism of giving groups ethical status, or rights to capabilities. Group-level analysis of inequalities in health capabilities must be done, but it has to be driven by concern for the capabilities of individuals within the groups. At the least, rather than denying groups rights, deny holism, or lay out a new theory about individualism in social science, this book attempts to elucidate a positive argument for an individual's right to CH. There is no question that the argument for the CH and CA more generally would benefit from giving more consideration to the philosophy of causation in the sciences as well as methodological individualism in

the social sciences. Studying the works of Rajeev Bhargava on individualism in social sciences, of Nancy Cartwright on causation, and
of Larry Temkin on individualistic inequality would be a good place
to start (Temkin, 1993; Cartwright, 2007; Bhargava, 2008).

Aggregation

It is familiar in political philosophy or economics to see groups as
simply the aggregation of individuals, and the problem that follows
from that tends to be about choosing between efficiency and equity.
Human health concerns can indeed be framed in terms of efficiency or
equity as economists frame it. Or, as philosophers, starting with John
Taurek have done, framed the problem in terms of whether numbers
count in deciding whether to help one group of individuals that is
larger than another (Taurek, 1977). The issue of trade-offs or aggregation cannot be avoided even by the CA.

Even the approach advocated by Nussbaum, and the present argument for the CH, which sees a set of capabilities as pre-political entitlements belonging to every human being cannot avoid the issue.
Nussbaum says emphatically, in those situations where every individual
does not have all of the basic capabilities, it must be seen as justice not
being done. Some would resist such an argument and point to the
necessity to rank capabilities as resources are limited everywhere and
must be efficiently allocated. Nussbaum would probably respond by
comparing the CHCs to basic rights and reply that no one argues for
trade-offs when it comes to basic constitutional rights. Such basic rights
are constrained only in relation to the exercise of other basic rights, but
a right is never completely denied for another. Similar is the case for
basic capabilities and aggregation of capabilities across individuals.
The CHCs cannot be ranked but must all be provided. Where some
cannot be fully provided up to the threshold level, then it must be seen
as justice not yet being done. Where there is a conflict between two
rights, or two right choices, Nussbaum contends that it is a tragic choice,
and, in the first instance, compels the consideration of how such a situation has come about and how to prevent it occurring in the future.

There is another aggregation problem that arises at the population
level. Creating a supportive external social environment for individual
health capabilities often entails affecting the mean-levels of behaviour
in the population, their cultural norms. Changing the legal age for
drinking, harsher penalties for drunk driving, making condoms freely

available and without embarrassment are examples of efforts to change the social norms. However, the individuals who are most vulnerable to impairments are often the hardest to reach. The majority of efforts to change the social norms do not reach individuals who may be isolated by social, economic and even physical and psychological constraints. Moreover, addressing the vulnerabilities of these few individuals does not affect the level of risk to the entire population. That is, the number of individuals who will face a small risk of impairment in the general population can outnumber the individuals in the high-risk group or the 'tail-end' of the population. Public health programmes that aim to maximize the health achievements of individuals are faced with particularly wicked aggregation or efficiency problems. Should they improve the health of a large number of people a little bit, or focus on the individuals that are the most likely to be impaired?

The CA and the argument for the CH reorient that choice and the moral function of public health. The respect for the equal dignity of every human being means that consequential evaluation of actions to maximize health capabilities cannot stop short of addressing the constraints of those most difficult to reach. Improving the capabilities of the many does not make up for others not having their minimal or threshold level of capabilities commensurate with human dignity. To neglect the health concerns of those in the tails – the most likely to be impaired, hardest to reach and most expensive to help – would be to treat them as second-class citizens, as people who do not have equal dignity. Despite the possibility of producing more health or health capabilities by focusing on the general population, the duty to show equal respect to each citizen entails protecting, promoting and restoring the CH of the those individuals most vulnerable or severely impaired.

Biology and group rights

Another issue that has not often been considered is that identifying and mitigating the determinants and consequences of health constraints in individuals can have repercussions for various groups to which the individuals belong. For example, if a genetic attribute is identified as a risk factor, then individuals who are identified with that attribute, their families and others related to those individuals may find themselves facing discrimination. Or, indeed, as experience with HIV/AIDS around the world has evidenced, when certain individuals are identified as being at high risk, various groups they belong to become the target of social discrimination. At the same time, biomedical research can often have repercussions for groups, while researchers deal respectfully with individual interests.

For example, collecting genetic material for databases can be garnered through consent from individuals, but the methods of handling biological materials may violate group beliefs and practices. The creation of 'immortalized' cell lines may be anathema to shared group beliefs. Or, interestingly, biomedical research into the genetic make up of a group of individuals may reveal information that contradicts shared understandings of lineage or place of origin that are central to group identity practices. The variety of ways in which addressing the health concerns of individuals can impact the shared beliefs and practices of groups once again highlights the possibility of groups having rights to capabilities. Or would the argument that groups can have claims only because of the moral concern for individuals within the group work here too?

Groups and borders

The analysis of health at the social group level is one of the most significant achievements in the field of public health. Despite the ferocious academic debates in epidemiology regarding the sustainability of the individual level bio-medical model in light of the population level analysis, there is much to be gained from making use of population health analysis. However, one of the interesting aspects of population level analysis is the question of where to draw the borders of the population or the place where the health issue is taking place (Trostle, 2004; Venkatapuram, 2006).

This challenge becomes more pressing for the CA, given that the conception of health as the CH advocated here is a species-wide notion. For most epidemiologists, the largest population group is the nation-state. But national borders have been arbitrarily drawn, nations have been divided and others have been unified. It might be simple to use national borders to assess the capabilities of individuals, as the UN Human Development Report does presently. But that does not mean that intervention to improve capabilities will necessarily be most effective at the national level. Individual capabilities can be affected by the social conditions including the features of the family, community, nation-state and global geographical region. There are many ways to group individuals. And the type of health issue will probably identify which grouping provides the most robust explanation and required intervention.

Conclusion

This chapter has aimed to introduce some of the group aspects of health concerns. In particular, it has tried to show how analysis of social group differences in order to identify social determinants of health should not automatically mean that groups themselves should be the primary focus of justice. The discussion has also tried to point to the difference between identifying the causes of the incidence rates of health constraints in a population and the causes of individual impairment. This was in order to point out that addressing incidence rates may involve recognizing the features of groups and possibly such a concept as group capability.

The brief discussion also touched on aggregation and how the CA, particularly the argument for the CHCs and CH, might handle an allocation decision that pits the capabilities of the many against the one or the few. Social determinants of health research demonstrate that health capabilities and functionings of individuals are really bound up in processes that extend much beyond an individual's own volitional choices and agency. The argument for the CH reflects this by asserting the interdependence of CHCs as well as the interdependence of individuals. Yet, it is still uncertain whether inter-dependent individuals with shared ends constitute something more than just individuals. In any case, group level analysis of the CH is something that is aligned with the individual entitlement to the CH because it reflects the moral concern for individuals belonging to the groups.

7

The Capability to be Healthy and Global Justice

In this chapter, I discuss what every human being's moral entitlement to the CH means for social interactions and institutions functioning across national or political borders. This chapter should, perhaps, have been the first chapter in the book rather than the last because the primary motivation behind the present work was to identify what moral claims or rights individuals across societies have in regard to their health and longevity. That search or question arose from participating in the agitation for health-related claims in developed countries during the early years of the HIV/AIDS epidemic as well as from attempting to address the high burden of preventable impairments and premature mortality in developing countries, in which HIV/AIDS again played a role. I assumed, perhaps too simplistically, that if individuals in various corners of the world were facing the same health risks and constraints, and societies everywhere were dealing with their citizens in an abusive manner, and governments seem to come and go, there must be a plausible path to identifying entitlements of individual human beings outside national borders and legal structures.

We often judge societies and laws as being just or unjust. And in order to determine whether a society is just or unjust, we must be drawing on ideas external to what is agreed or practised within those countries. What could those ideas be? Many individuals are drawn to international human rights law because it is meant to be such a supranational source of rights, and increasingly responsibilities, of human beings. But how do the rights get onto the list in the first place? How do we decide the conflict of rights? Or, what do we do when we disagree vehemently with the majority of the expert legal opinion that there is no such thing as a human right to health and instead, only a human right to healthcare?[1]

Therein lies the difficulty in trying to bring together the indignation and sense of injustice about aspects of impairments and mortality in different societies on the one hand with the intellectual and academic problem of conceptualizing justice across national borders on the other hand. Global justice is often the last chapter in a book, sometimes an afterthought, or presented as a necessary gesture. This is because over the past fifty years or so since political philosophy has been revitalized, the most actively developed area of social justice philosophy has been based on the social contract tradition. This in turn, was a reaction to the previously dominant philosophy of utilitarianism. The consequence of this is that within the social contract tradition, or in debates between social contract theorists and utlitarians, justice is implicitly understood as something that exists only within a community of individuals who are part of the social contract. Global justice, as a result, becomes a question about whether justice applies outside the social contract, and if so, what does that entail?

And so, the last chapter often gestures towards what may or may not be required outside the social contract that was the main focus of the book. Philosophers may feel required to make such an effort because just as it is implausible for a theory of justice not to treat individuals with equal concern and respect within a social contract, it increasingly seems implausible to not show at least some sort of moral concern for human beings outside one's national borders. This is due to a range of factors including the visible effects of intensified globalization, growing awareness of the complicity of domestic institutions in the deprivations experienced by foreigners, the great imbalance in global negotiations on trade or environment, recognition of the longstanding impact of colonialism, and so forth.

Let me begin by presenting two arguments against justice producing any duties regarding the CH of individuals outside one's national borders, or global health justice more broadly. One argument moves from principles to practice. And the second moves in the opposite direction from practicalities to principles. Thomas Nagel writes in what is now considered to be a seminal essay on global justice that there is no such thing as justice across nations (Nagel, 2005). Nagel, reflecting a long history of thinkers, argues that a sovereign state is required to enforce or apply justice through institutions. Without such a sovereign global state or a world government, and it is uncertain whether that would in fact be such a good thing, the problems of human deprivations we may be concerned about in the world have to be dealt under some other moral principles, not under justice. So, under Nagel's reasoning, we might speak of the right to CH within a domestic sphere where there is a sovereign government capable of shaping and moving social institutions, with 'coercive authority'. But, there are no duties from justice to address the various dimensions of the CH outside of national borders because there is no global state.

A parallel line of argument is presented by Angus Deaton in his evaluation of the morality of addressing health inequalities. Rightly giving more consideration to the causes of impairments and mortality than is usually given in the literature on health justice Deaton, nevertheless, takes a position against international duties to address preventable ill-health and mortality in other (developing) countries. This duty, he argues, is primarily the job of national governments, which currently seem either unable or uninterested in fulfilling that duty. And foreign governments, NGOs, or philanthropists going into alleviate impairments and preventable mortality can actually make the situation worse. Deaton writes:

> International health inequalities cannot be eliminated without the construction of well-functioning domestic healthcare systems that provide to the citizens of poor countries the preventative, pre- and post-natal and maternal care that is routine in rich countries. These systems cannot be constructed from the outside, but require domestic state capacity, institutions and responsibility to citizens that is often missing in poor countries, and that may well actually be undermined by large financial flows from outside. (Deaton, 2011, p. 17)

He does not deny the manifest injustice in the impairments and premature mortality in poor countries, or that first-world knowledge has significantly alleviated burdens of ill-health, or that international actions can continue to do more with regard to health constraints in poor countries. Rather, speaking against cosmopolitan philosophers who identify certain duties to all human beings irrespective of national borders, Deaton argues that the practicalities are against them; they would be doing more harm than good by going in to build targeted health programmes. Deaton asserts that most of the ill-health and premature mortality would be effectively addressed by well-functioning healthcare systems, which entails a functioning national government taking an interest, and applying principles of justice through social institutions. And so Deaton, like Nagel, sees justice as something that requires a sovereign, functioning state government taking action through institutions locally. So there are both arguments from theoretical principles and practical evaluation of health issues against global duties from justice to address the CH of human beings outside one's national borders.

For many years, philosophers were quite content with discussing the intellectual puzzles arising within an idealized world of a single society or simply, domestic justice. But the events in the real world have been too significant, if not world changing, to be ignored. Global financial meltdowns, climate change, infectious diseases and transnational social movements claiming to be fighting injustice across countries present compelling questions about what is the right thing to do about the well-being or quality of life of human beings living in countries across the world. Reasoning about global justice, for many who come from the social contract tradition, is seen to mean perhaps, extending the reasoning about justice domestically to those outside the social contract, to those human beings living outside national and political borders. The theoretical social contract and real-world national borders overlap. And as these discussions about how to extend social justice to the global sphere proceed, there is in the background the history and philosophy of human rights. Most of that philosophy, as I mentioned in Chapter 5, concludes that human rights are in need of coherent theoretical foundations.

As Daniels puts it, 'Rights are not moral fruits that spring up from the bare earth, fully ripened, without cultivation' (Daniels, 2008, p. 15). Whether moral rights or human rights, rights need to be grounded in ethical reasoning. So to reconcile social justice philosophy with the real world of multiple societies and the body of human rights law we are looking for a theory of global justice from which we can 'cultivate' rights for every human being. Theorizing about global justice while ignoring human rights would be hazardous, given that they do reflect ethical ideas developed through reasoning across societies; the corpus of human rights law represents something important about our global social and political culture. An approach or theory or social justice in the modern world needs to account for multiple and interdependent societies as well as the enduring consensus regarding the ideas articulated by international human rights law.

From the start, the CA has been a theory distinct from theories of the social contract tradition. In the case of Nussbaum, her theory explicitly starts with a list of entitlements that every human being has wherever we find them. And, in turn, the central argument of this book has been that every human being has an entitlement to a CH, a meta-capability to a cluster of basic capabilities and functionings, each to a level that is commensurate with equal human dignity in the modern world. So while the CA derives the claims to capabilities, or to a specific list of basic capabilities, from the fundamental social values of freedoms and equal dignity, the CA also asserts that such entitlements belong to every human being wherever we find them. The metric of justice in the CA is the social bases of capabilities, and the distribution rule is up to the level that is equitable. In Nussbaum's theory, claims are to the social bases of capabilities up to a level commensurate with equal human dignity. While Nussbaum identifies these claims for basic capabilities as arising out of the dignity of the human animal understood as a needy and sociable being with capacity to reason, I have, in essence, wrapped around the basic capabilities, the definition of human health. Health or the CH produces moral claims for supportive social conditions wherever we find human beings. From this perspective, justice is not something that resides only in government powers, or in ideal social institutions, but in the capabilities of human beings. The focus on human capabilities rather than on institutions is a central difference between social contract theories and the CA with far reaching implications, particularly for global justice. Making sense of such a statement may require a brief description of the philosophy of cosmopolitanism.

Cosmopolitanism

Whether referring to peoples, societies or nation-states, Rawls and others base their conception of social justice on the social contract tradition that conceives of individuals as having distinctly different rights and obligations within their societal borders versus outside. Taken to an extreme, this 'relational-statist' position – though no particular theory or individual advocates the extreme – contends that there are absolutely no moral rights and responsibilities to individuals or other entities outside one's own societal borders (Sangiovanni, 2007). Justice does not exist in the space or relations between societies. At the other end of the spectrum, there is the extreme 'cosmopolitan' position – which only a few individuals advocate – which asserts that there exist the same moral rights and responsibilities between all individuals irrespective of societal borders (Singer, 1972; Beitz, 1988; Caney, 2005). At this end of the spectrum, national borders simply have no moral significance.

The history of cosmopolitanism is long and appears to be traceable across many ancient civilizations. In particular, the cosmopolitan thinking of many modern and early philosophers is traced to ancient Greece and the Stoics (Brown and Held, 2010). Three normative tenets form the core of cosmopolitan thought. First, individual human beings are the ultimate units of moral concern. Second, this moral concern attaches to every human being equally. And third, this concern applies to every human being wherever we find them in the world. Different theorists take different paths to get to the point of asserting the equal moral concern for every human being. And they differ on what that entails in terms of social institutions. That is, some would argue that social institutions are a necessary part of realizing even cosmopolitan justice. Therefore, there must be much thought given to what sort of global social institutions could exist that would be able to realize equal concern and respect through social institutions.

Others contend that justice does not need the ideal specification of global institutions nor does it require government institutions to alleviate injustice outside of national borders (O'Neill, 2000; Sen, 2009). Justice can be created or extinguished, increased or lessened, in the quality of people's lives, their capabilities. In any case, while there may be differences among cosmopolitan thinkers about the locus of justice, the basic materials of cosmopolitan thought are the commitment to individual human beings, equality and universality.

Despite the landscape in the global justice debates being painted as disagreement between the relational-statist versus the cosmopolitan positions, most of the well-known arguments in the debates take a middle-ground position. There are obligations to both fellow-nationals and foreigners, but there are stricter and broader obligations to fellow-nationals and for different reasons. The debates are largely about the nuances of the theoretical structures that defend a position closer to one side or another of the spectrum. Rawls' conception of global justice, for instance, is clearly on the relational-statist side of the spectrum. He advocates a two-stage process which begins with a domestic social contract between individuals, and then a global contract between societies. This second stage of the contract identifies some principles governing the interactions between societies including some basic duties to assist or intervene in other societies. For example, he argues that there are duties to assist such as 'insisting on human rights' in poor countries, which he calls burdened societies, in order to engender good government and to prevent famines. In comparison to the broad range of rights and duties within the domestic sphere, these duties to assist seem fairly minimal and they in fact may not be the same as duties of justice. This is particularly true if one follows the line of reasoning that justice can only apply where there is either a coercive state apparatus or a system of mutual cooperation.

As I discussed in the Introduction, many aspects of theorizing about social justice erase concerns about some central aspects of individuals' well-being such as their health, and also lead to various moral errors. Also, such theoretical structures can produce conceptions of social justice that seem perfectly coherent given the traditions and assumptions but seem hollow in light of the greatest injustices occurring in the world. This was the case with Norman Daniels' first argument on health justice. He extended the best available non-utilitarian theory of social justice in order to address health concerns. But, this best available theory imagined the world as if it contained only one society. Moreover, this single society and the social contract on which it is based is predicated on the existence of moderate scarcity of resources, a rough equality in physical and mental powers of members, mutual disinterest and the coexistence of persons at the same time in a geographical territory (Rawls, 1971, pp. 126–130).

These assumptions essentially erase the possibility of applying justice, and the relevance of theorizing about justice, to most human beings living in the world. Rawls' theory of justice erases both human impairments and mortality in theorizing about social justice, and erases the societies where health issues are the most acute and persistent. So we come back again to the tension between theoretical structures used in philosophical arguments about justice and the demand from human dignity that theories of justice should be relevant to the central concerns of human beings. It seems implausible that one could choose to work with a theory such as that of Rawls without recognizing that it erases the moral worry about the health impairments and premature mortality risk experienced by the vast majority of the human species and that it is restricted in being able to provide guidance in a world where human beings live in numerous societies, and with remarkable diversity in health and longevity. I will return shortly to discussing how there are some rare and notable attempts to extend social contracts, such as that advanced by Rawls, to the entire human species. More presently, I want to highlight why the capabilities approach and argument for the CH do better at global justice from the start.

CA and global justice

The CA expresses the view that a theory of justice has to be fully aware of extra-societal ethical issues from the beginning (Sen, 2005, 2009). When a theory of social justice begins with the individual human being as the primary moral agent, and in order to show equal respect and concern to every human being, the theory has to recognize the important differences in the abilities of persons to pursue life plans. These differences arise from the independent effects and interactions of their internal physical and mental features, 'conversion skills' and their external social and physical conditions. The CA does not exclude considering the possibility that these sources of differences in individuals could be negatively or positively affected by factors from outside national borders. Nor does the CA sidestep or deny moral responsibilities in relation to one's actions negatively influencing the well-being or capabilities of individuals living outside of one's own national borders.

However, while the former empirical point and the latter ethical point may be uncontroversial, the CA stands apart from other leading social justice theories in explicitly identifying positive obligations to help realize capabilities of human beings outside of one's own national borders. The nature and scope of the obligations can vary according to the social bases of the causal pathways of the capabilities and functionings of the foreigners. The source of such moral obligations, for Nussbaum, arises out of the respect for the equal human dignity and moral worth of every human being. Remember, human dignity is a source of claims wherever it is found. For Sen, it lies in the value of freedom and effective power of agents – in their possession of power effectively to nurture, protect, remedy or restore the capabilities and freedoms of individuals. Unlike other arguments for social justice, the CA does not need to relax any assumptions or make theoretical compromises that integrate the 'non-ideal' considerations of the international system. The CA takes all human beings as they are, and the world as it is, in order to identify and evaluate the ethical claims and duties of individuals across national and political borders. The focus on human capabilities has resulted in theoretical structures of the CA expressing central cosmopolitan values of humanity, equality and universality.

As an alternative to a largely or completely closed social contract approach to social and global justice, the CA advocates two methods of reasoning that resist looking only within societies when reasoning about justice. That is, methods of reasoning about what duties one has to foreigners but also in reasoning about justice more broadly. One method of reasoning is to try to take the view of an 'impartial spectator' when evaluating the social arrangements of a society. While impartiality runs through the work of many philosophers, Sen advocates for Adam Smith's conception of impartiality as it seems to allow judgements of disinterested individuals from other societies into social decision-making in the domestic context (Sen, 2005, 2009, pp . 44–46, 149–152). The second approach is to recognize a set of minimum social entitlements for every human being wherever they are found.

On the one hand, the impartial observer would be able to look at a situation like that of Daniels' dyslexic individual in an illiterate society and be able to reason that just because the majority is illiterate or, indeed, dying at a young age, does not mean these social facts determine the moral claims to a good life for this individual. In so far as an entire society can share a common sympathy or indeed a common hatred as the case may be, it does not mean that whatever is the shared norm is necessarily morally legitimate. On the other hand, by upholding a basic metric and a rule – a set of basic capabilities and functionings at sufficient thresholds commensurate with equal human dignity in the modern world – across every human being, we can reason across societies about what minimal justice requires in regard to individuals.

What Sen, Nussbaum and other CA advocates argue is that within a particular society realizing social justice entails ensuring that individuals have equitable capabilities, particularly with respect to some basic capabilities. In societies where governments are unable to ensure basic capabilities or locations where there is no functioning state, the duties to assist in protecting and nurturing basic capabilities belong to a range of actors. Sen provides the reasoning that duties fall on any agent that possesses the effective power to alleviate the deprivations of others because possessing the effective power creates an obligation to at least consider taking action to do so (Sen, 2009, pp. 205–207, 372–376). Nussbaum grounds her justification for the duties of each person to ensure the basic capabilities of others in the recognition of equal dignity and the good of shared sociability.

However, capabilities advocates, while identifying fairly stringent duties to assist individuals across borders, do not minimize the importance of sovereignty or national borders. The obligations to support the entitlements to basic capabilities of every human being should not be seen as being immediately overwhelming, to the point of undermining the identity or sovereignty of a nation. Indeed, sovereignty must be respected from the perspective of the CA because it is an expression of individual freedom and self-determination in creating a state. Individuals may reasonably delegate their obligations to institutions for a range of good reasons including those of collective action problems, to fairly divide the duties, because of limited capacity, and to limit the responsibilities from erasing an individual's personal life (Nussbaum, 2006, pp. 307–308). So, if Deaton's empirical assertion that most of impairments and premature mortality in poor countries are due to the lack of infrastructure, then the CA would see helping to build that infrastructure as part of showing equal respect. When governments show disinterest, then the moral demands from people's CH require supporting non-governmental and other institutions to address the various dimensions of the CH.

Health and cosmopolitan justice

The conception of CH as a species-wide entitlement is central to its extension of the CA. However, such a conception also has significant implications for any theory of social justice that intends to distribute health, or more accurately, the social bases of health. In Chapter 1 I rejected the prevailing notion of health as species typical functioning and argued that a conception of health is coherent only as a fully ethical idea that is applicable to every member of the human species. Health is a capability to achieve a cluster of basic capabilities. The components of the cluster are identified through free-standing ethical reasoning aiming for overlapping consensus across societies.

The consequence for this, I would argue, is that any theory of justice that seeks to guarantee the social bases of health, using this coherent idea of health, becomes a cosmopolitan theory of justice. Perhaps I should sharpen this point further. Theories of justice which continue to use the Boorsean concept of health as the absence of disease or other notions of health that are not coherent are building their theories on broken ideas. The *most coherent* way to conceptualize health is to see it as a cluster of basic capabilities commensurate with equal human dignity in the contemporary world. So, when the CH is placed in the 'what' or primary goods space of any theory of justice, it explodes it into a cosmopolitan theory.

If health were defined as a purely descriptive idea, as Daniels does in using the label 'species typical functioning' or a socially relative concept, then indeed there would be no obligation to provide the social bases of CH to foreigners as there would be for those inside the social contract/national borders. But because health is not a purely objective idea, and though it may be a concept that is socially relative above the thresholds, there is a central core concept of health that is an ethical idea pertaining to the dignity of the human being. Respecting the equal dignity of every human being means ensuring a sufficient threshold of the CH of individuals that is commensurate with equal human dignity of those inside and outside of one's societal borders. The lack of respect for the dignity of human beings outside national borders undermines the dignity of members inside the borders (Margalit, 1996). Responsibilities of diverse agents, however, will vary according to their capacities and relationship to the causes, consequences, persistence, levels and distribution of the CH achievements and failures as well as possibilities for social action.

Self-determination and health

In following through a social-contract/relational-statist approach to health and justice across societies, such a perspective holds that it is just that an individual's life prospects are relative to their society. That is to say, there is nothing about justice that relates to the differences in health and longevity between nations, but only about differences within nations. Such reasoning follows from seeing the value of respecting a society's or community's social values and other shared features. Some philosophers also seek to apply that same notion of respect or neutrality to the economic and material conditions of a society. Just as some philosophers may find it important that social justice claims related to an individual's life prospects are evaluated in relation the opportunity range shaped by social values, other philosophers argue that an individual's life prospects should also be relative to the opportunity range determined by the society's level of development and wealth. The level of economic development is seen as being similar to culture and shared sympathies (Pogge, 1989; Rawls, 1999).

One way of reaching this understanding is to see a society's level of development and wealth as being determined wholly by domestic factors such as the social and political culture of its citizens. The level of social and economic development is itself an expression of social values and thus it is reasonable to evaluate the justness of social arrangements by comparing the achievements of individuals with what other individuals are able to achieve in that society. What this means with respect to health, if it is taken to its logical conclusion, is that an individual's health is compared to the health of other co-nationals. So, for example, if the average or 'normal' life expectancy in a society is twenty-five years, then any individual in that society would have claims to an opportunity range for twenty-five years of life.

Alternatively, it could be argued that the individual has a claim to the social basis of reaching twenty-five years of life because achieving a twenty-five year lifespan is thought to be a valuable thing for every member of that society. So living for twenty-five years could be valuable because it is instrumentally useful to equality of opportunity to achieve the normal range of life plans or because of its inherent value to a member of that society. In the former example, twenty-five years is the standard because that is the most common and represents normality. In the latter, twenty-five years could have been chosen because there is something valuable about having the same longevity as others, or about living for close to or exactly twenty-five years of life. In this way health is both a product of social values and culture as well as an expression of social values and culture.

Normal opportunity range

Norman Daniels seems to takes such a position in both his initial and newly revised argument. He provides the example that a person with dyslexia would not have any social justice claims for assistance even from domestic institutions in a society which is largely illiterate (Daniels, 2008, p. 45). If the most common range of life plans of a society does not value literacy, then dyslexia does not constrain achieving a fair share of that range. Therefore, the individual has no claims to social support for alleviating dyslexia because to be literate is not part of the normal opportunity range. Daniels gives no value to the possibility that literacy is a good thing for a human being, irrespective of the literacy of the surrounding population. Nor does Daniels acknowledge that literacy is an inherent and instrumentally valuable functioning for a human being in the contemporary world. As societies are becoming more integrated, it seems reasonable to think that being literate will be instrumentally even more valuable in the future. Of course, given this line of argument about dyslexia, Daniels also has to contend that individuals will only have entitlements to the most common range of life expectancy values as well. It is quite ironic that domestically Daniels attempts to guarantee as expansive a range of life prospects as possible for individuals – given their corrected talents and motivations – by not guaranteeing their chosen share of the normal range of life plans only but also their *fair* share of the full range. Yet, internationally, he is willing to accept that the normal range of life plans in certain societies will be quite narrow, not because the individual chose them, or because of their talents and skills, but because of what is most common in the society.

Irrespective of whether the level of economic and social development of a society reflects the social values and culture of that society, identifying entitlements based on what is commonly achieved in that particular society is unsatisfying. It does makes sense that because individuals living in rich countries continually push at the upper boundaries of longevity, individuals in such societies should be able to make claims for the social bases of the most commonly achieved life plans, or even the most commonly achieved states of well-being. Their fair share can be expected to help them achieve the upper bounds of human longevity because the most common values are at the upper end of the spectrum. There is no need to make any kind of argument in these societies that individuals have claims to achieve the upper bounds of human longevity because the most common longevity values are already at the high bounds. And the notion of equality of opportunity meshes well with the statistically typical achieved values. What sense would there be of ensuring the equality of opportunity to achieve a lifespan that is currently impossible, or a lifespan that is so low that it is virtually guaranteed for every individual without any social inputs? Equality of opportunity only makes sense when the opportunities are valuable.

However, imagine the case that economic development resulted in dramatic decreases in human longevity for the entire population. Then it would almost be guaranteed that the arguments for the equality of opportunity to achieve the most common values versus opportunity to achieve the upper bound values would exist separately. That is, if poverty were to protect and improve human longevity, it would be likely that individuals in rich countries would want to switch from having the equality of opportunity to achieve 'normal range' or most common values of longevity to having the equality of opportunity to achieve the global, upper bound values. And they would surely mobilize social institutions to realize that principle. The argument for the equality of opportunity to achieve a fair share of the normal range of life prospects obfuscates the underlying value given to living a lifespan as long as possible. Such an argument is acceptable only in countries or regions of the world where there is high longevity.

In contrast, an argument for the CH links the levels of health and longevity to equal human dignity. And respect for human dignity does not entail bringing down the longevity of those in rich countries, or of narrowing their normal opportunity range, but the provision of the social bases for improving the CH of all human beings up to a level that puts people in the state of equal dignity with others. Such equal dignity is likely to be found when all human beings, all things considered, have the CH to achieve the highest average human functionings currently possible.

Two problems

At least two areas need greater exploration in the area of health and global/social justice. The first area concerns the reality that determinants of the health of individuals and populations are trans-national (O'Neill, 2002b). New and resurgent infectious diseases beginning with the HIV/AIDS epidemic in the 1980s, followed by SARS, avian flu, foot and mouth disease, multi-drug-resistant tuberculosis and others, have brought to the forefront how the increasing interconnectedness of societies also makes them more vulnerable to biological threats to life. For a multitude of man-made reasons, the rate at which new and resurgent infectious diseases affect human populations has been steadily increasing over the past three decades. Indeed, such vulnerability to biological threats through interconnectedness was thoroughly apparent in the spread of the bubonic plague that started in China before entering Europe in the fourteenth century.

Though the history of infectious diseases and human populations show the consequences of both ever-growing settled populations and interactions between such settled communities, it is hard to ignore the fact that the determinants of health across trans-national borders are not just infectious biological organisms. Social and material factors also move across borders. The social and economic relationships between societies have historically had both negative and positive impact on the health of individuals and populations. Sometimes the critics of contemporary globalization or colonialism underplay the benefits to health of interconnectedness.

In contrast, negative examples are aplenty. For example, the European settlers in the American colonies, in some cases unknowingly, and in some cases purposefully, altered the social and material conditions which resulted in the extinction of various native populations. That is, aside from killing them simply by using guns, their continual annexation of land and denial of access to traditional ways of sustenance resulted in dramatic increases in mortality and impairments.

At the same time, the wealth from trade as well as knowledge from other societies have improved the health and life expectancy of many European countries. Also, increasing forms and speed of communication have allowed citizens of developing countries to reap health benefits just from information such as that on nutrition, sanitation or biological threats. The health benefits and burdens resulting from the longstanding relationships between human communities are undeniable even if there is disagreement about which benefit and burden has been greater for a given society.

The historical evidence of the positive and negative effects of trans-national interactions on the health of individuals and populations militates against the idea that there is no global society or that human societies are mutually independent entities. Though there may well be significant disagreements about when the processes of interconnected-ness between societies really became established in which parts of the world, there can be little doubt that contemporary societies are and will become even more inter-related. If nothing else, the rapid spread across national borders of infectious diseases through human interaction evidences the shared vulnerabilities arising from being human beings, and the necessity to coordinate a response across the human community to mitigate the vulnerability.

Conversely, global society can be made up from the shared vulner-ability of human beings to biological threats that arise from interac-tions, and the necessity to coordinate an appropriate response. From there, it becomes easier to see that it is not only infectious biological agents but social and material determinants that also require regulat-ing. As a result of the ever more increasing interdependence of human societies across the world, addressing the shared vulnerabilities result-ing from the common features of human beings can be a source of cooperation across societies in contrast to establishing mutual deter-rence principles against aggression from other societies. The mutual recognition of the vulnerabilities to premature death and impairments as a result of human interactions within and across societies forms the basis of recognizing a global society of individual human beings, rather than one of national states (Turner, 2006).

The processes of trans-national interactions which transform mate-rial and social conditions of societies that then influence the mortality and impairment burden of individuals and populations are easily rec-ognizable in many contemporary societies. There are many who argue that increased economic development through greater participation in the global economy will result directly in the improved longevity and quality of life of populations. Such a causal relationship may some-times be true depending on the choice of economic policies, as evi-denced by the varied experiences of China, India, Japan and other South-East Asian countries.

The opposite can also be the case as evidenced by the rise in prevent-able mortality and impairments in Russia after economic liberalization programmes. In light of both the vulnerabilities engendered by societal interconnectedness as well as the possible benefits, there are many ethical issues that arise in regard to the terms of trans-societal social cooperation.

In regard to health, there is a pressing concern to identify the terms of trans-national interactions in order to mitigate the biological as well as the social determinants which undermine the CH of individuals and populations of all societies. If the equality of opportunity to achieve a fair share of life plans is a basic entitlement in a particular society, or the CH is an entitlement, then ensuring such an entitlement would require engaging with the broad spectrum of agents which influence determinants originating from within and outside the national borders.

The second area of concern is the question of what claims individuals can make to agents outside of their national borders when the basic social institutions within are either purposefully constraining their CH or lack the resources or knowledge to provide the social basis of the capability. Or indeed, the basic social institutions are only partially existent if at all. In times of acute crisis that may overwhelm the capacity of a society's institutions to respond adequately, agents outside the national borders may be motivated by beneficence to provide assistance in the form of material goods and other technological resources. But what about the low-level endemic constraints on the health capability of individuals and populations during non-emergencies? Can claims to support health capability still only appeal to beneficence? As I stated at the beginning of the chapter, Angus Deaton asserts that in such cases intervening may actually do more harm as the primary cause of the ill-health and mortality is the lack of a health system.

It may seem at first that in countries with the highest magnitude of preventable mortality and impairments what is needed to improve the health capability of individuals is material resources. Improved nutrition, adequate sanitation, better housing conditions, vaccinations, education and so forth would dramatically relieve the constraints on the capability of individuals to be healthy. But a more thorough examination of even the most basic causal pathways to health in the poorest of countries would show that the causal pathway includes both material goods and social conditions. Even what seems to be a purely resource issue such as improving the rates of infant mortality through the provision of vaccinations requires addressing the social conditions in which mothers are situated. The availability of the vaccine in a particular locale has to be matched with the social conditions which allow mothers to be aware of its availability and efficacy, as well as the freedom to move physically to access the resource for their infant.

Indeed, the availability of resources such as vaccinations lead to thinking that the CH of individuals could improve significantly simply with the provision of material goods at a certain point in time. The 'silver bullet' approach that is focused on providing goods to alleviate immediate threats to life or provide life-long immunity can have significant impact but only with respect to those specific threats. Ensuring that an individual has the capability of living a normal length of life and avoid impairments requires a supportive social and material environment over the life course. In light of this, individuals still have moral claims against agents outside of their national borders when their health capability is being maliciously constrained by domestic agents, or their society's institutions are simply incapable of adequately addressing the various dimensions of the entitlement to the CH.

Kingdom of capabilities

There is a loss when ethical reasoning loses sight of the liberal principle of each person as an end. Even though utilitarian aggregation has been largely shunned since Rawls, the global justice debates currently use aggregate analysis that looks far too similar to utilitarian analysis. The most prominent example can be seen in Charles Jones' argument for achieving global justice, which entails protecting certain basic human rights (Jones, 1999). He argues that if there are any basic human rights, then there are basic rights to food, clothing, education and so forth. But his argument for ensuring such rights is that they will improve overall, global welfare. Despite the use of the rhetoric of basic human rights, it is rule-utilitarianism par excellence.

Philosophers who start with peoples and nations as primary agents of global justice or who carelessly slip into group analysis when evaluating global inequalities compromise the basic starting principle of the distinctness of human beings. Nussbaum, for example, criticizes Rawls for his willingness or toleration of the violence against women by allowing for 'decent peoples' to be part of his global social contract rather than only liberal societies that treat every human being with equal respect. The emphasis on the necessity to be 'realistic' in the interactions with other societies and to be tolerant of the violation of individual dignity or similarly, be satisfied with improving aggregate indicators of well-being in other societies undermines the integrity of the arguments used to justify domestic theories of justice.

Conclusion

The identification of entitlements and duties of individuals irrespective of where they are in the global society places the CA on the cosmopolitan side of the global justice debates. The CA upholds all the basic tenets of cosmopolitanism. All members of the human species are the primary agents of social justice; they have equal human dignity, wherever they are in the world. A conception of global justice is built up from the individual and continually refers back to the capabilities of individuals. Justice lies not in ideal institutions or only in government institutions but in human capabilities. Basic capabilities understood as pre-political claims are paired with duties to a diverse set of agents, not only within national borders but across national borders. By examining more closely the causal components of a person's capability to be healthy, the distribution of CH, the persistence over generations, levels, the differential experience and possible social remedies, we will be to identify the relevant agent. And we will be able to identify whether the duty is positive, negative or intermediary with regard to protecting, sustaining, promoting or restoring the CH of individuals.

Conclusion

In this concluding chapter, I restate the basic argument for the CH. Then I highlight some of the theoretical contributions of this work. I hope that some of the contributions will be seen to be worthy of further examination by CA theorists as they affect the CA more broadly. I finish the chapter and book by discussing two important limitations and look towards the next set of questions. As I said in the Introduction, this book is the first instalment of a long-term project to put health at the centre of the theory and practical evaluation of social justice.

Health justice, as I have argued in this book, begins from a conception of human health as a person's abilities to achieve or exercise a cluster of basic human activities and opportunities. These 'beings and doings' are in turn specified through ethical reasoning about what constitutes a minimal conception of a life with equal human dignity in the modern world. Health is a meta-capability, an overarching capability to achieve or exercise a cluster of inter-related and basic capabilities to be and do things. This conception rejects the notion of health as the absence of disease, and advocates a positive conception of health as a cluster of abilities to be and do things. Such a conception also avoids conflating health with total well-being by being limited to a core set of capabilities. The moral claim or entitlement to such a cluster of capabilities or health capability arises out of freedoms and equal human dignity as fundamental values no one could reasonably reject. Health is a kind of freedom that has both intrinsic and instrumental value. And health is human dignity; the dignity of human beings is reflected in their capabilities of achieving certain basic activities and opportunities. The basic capabilities and the CH are a minimum conception of human well-being worthy of the dignity of the human being.

Based on the template of Drèze and Sen's model of the general theory of malnutrition and social epidemiology, an individual's CH or potential health 'beings and doings' are created by the interaction between (1) an individual's internal biological needs or features that change over the life cycle, (2) social conditions including extant material resources such as healthcare, (3) physical environment and (4) her agency or conversion skills; her physical and mental skills to 'convert' her own endowments and needs, and external social and physical conditions into health functionings. In purely descriptive terms, the failure to achieve certain health 'beings and doings' such as living a normal length of lifespan or avoiding impairments can be explained in terms of having a constrained set of 'beings and doings' due to the independent and interactive effects of the four determinants. The ultimate constraint is death.

Original arguments

While putting forward an interdisciplinary argument for an entitlement to a health capability, or right to health, the seven chapters presented some original contributions to the capability theory literature. In response to the ambiguous nature of health claims and the deference to medical science and health statistics in the CA, I argued for a conception of health as a capability to achieve a cluster of basic capabilities and functionings. This conception of health is not vulnerable to the longstanding criticisms against disease-centred notions of health, and links the CA to the state of the art debates in philosophy of health and medicine. The book also presented an analytical causal model of a human capability as being created by the independent and interactive determinants of biological endowments and needs, external environmental conditions, social conditions and conversion skills. This phenomenological account of capability is then integrated with epidemiological models allowing for the possibility of both social and natural scientists to work together in identifying the various dimensions of human capabilities including the causes, distributions, constraints, persistence, differential experiences and so forth. Furthermore, Sen and Drèze's entitlement analysis of famines and social epidemiological analyses are brought together to show how individual and population level explanations can be integrated.

I argued for a capability based theory of health causation and distribution. It integrates the individual level biomedical model with social determinants research and it goes beyond the focus on disease. Importantly, it allows the examination of the health issues of all human beings on a single plane of analysis, rather than the current situation where health issues of individuals in rich, poor and middle-income countries are evaluated under different frameworks each with their different background assumptions. The epidemiological theory of capabilities unifies the study of proximate determinants and supra-individual determinants as well as erases the distinction between rich and poor country issues. It has the possibility of being the framework for studying global health, just as the CA is seen as having the potential evaluating global well-being or quality of life.

The conception of health as capability and the theory of causation and distribution of health capability both provide independent support for a CH outside of the CA. This is important to note as the coherence of health as capability exists outside the CA and applicable to all discussions about health. Any theory of justice which seeks to address health claims will have to make use of the notion of health as a capability, or at least defend the conception of health being used given the Boorsean account or others like it are inadequate. Moreover, I illustrated how the moral claim to CH, and indeed any capability, can be understood as a 'cluster right'. Capabilities theorists should take notice of the advantage of fleshing out the right to a capability as a cluster of claims, powers, immunities and privileges. Doing so allows movement beyond discussions on whether rights to capabilities can only exist if and when there are correlative duty holders. Rights can also exist without identifiable duty holders and when they are not immediately fully realizable.

In Part III, an explicit analysis was presented of how a CH would fare against health equity principles, the health and human rights paradigm, and health claims from welfare or resource theories. I also evaluated Norman Daniels' revised Rawlsian theory of health justice and Shlomi Segall's health and luck egalitarian arguments from a capability perspective. Some basic ideas from social epidemiology and 'population health' are extended to the capabilities literature to argue that capability theory needs to clarify thinking about groups and their capabilities. Aside from taking the position that group level analysis does not necessarily mean that groups have ethical standing, I have offered no clear solution to the problem as to whether groups should be recognized as having moral claims to capabilities independently of the rights of individuals within the groups.

However, I identified some issues relating to groups and health that must be considered as well as some places to begin looking more concertedly at causation in social epidemiology, methodological individualism in social science and individualistic versus group inequalities. And in the final chapter, I argued against the position that there are no duties from justice to show equal concern and respect to human beings outside national borders. I showed how the CA upholds the basic tenets of cosmopolitanism, takes the view of individual capabilities as the locus of justice, and presented some weaknesses of other approaches. Lastly, it was argued that a coherent conception of health as a species-wide conception means that putting health claims in the 'primary goods space' of any distributive theory will tend to transform it into at least a minimally cosmopolitan theory of justice. Health of individuals everywhere in the world is determined by factors both inside and outside national borders. A basic commitment to the equal moral worth of every human being means that whoever falls within the scope of justice in any theory have to be held accountable for the effects of their actions on any and all other human beings in the world.

Limitations

As with any argument the one presented in this book also has limitations. There are two limitations that I want to identify in particular. The present book did not address the two distinct but related issues of aggregation and feasibility. Anyone studying or making public policy, including health policy, recognizes that policy decisions are made at the aggregate level. The 'real action' happens at the population level where resources are being allocated, where lives are being weighed. That is not to say that justice does not matter in the relations between individuals. Talking about individual entitlements is all good and right but, particularly in the domains of health, healthcare and public policy, the alternative ethical approaches present relatively clear frameworks to deal with aggregation and aggregation problems. That is, they have relatively clear distribution rules. A general theory of health justice needs to be able to guide reasoning, even when it is focused on health capabilities, on how to make decisions at the population level. Nussbaum argues that, in the first instance, there is no aggregation issue with the ten CHCs. Every individual is entitled to sufficient levels of each CHC. But, even as we move towards that goal, as Larry Temkin so insightfully illustrates, we need to think much harder about which scenario of inequality is better than another (Temkin, 1993).

And even Nussbaum recognizes that above the thresholds, or at the thresholds, different distributive principles should be considered (Nussbaum, 2000a). Sen, in contrast, advocates 'intersectionality' or partially theorized agreements. He fully expects that even after vested interests and personal priorities are removed from social decisions, there would still remain conflicting views on social priorities. Nevertheless, he maintains that the intersection or seeking commonality of the various rankings of justice will yield a partial ordering, making possible comparative judgements in many cases (Sen, 2009, pp. 104–105). Much more needs to be done in considering how to make aggregative decisions involving capabilities in general and health in particular. This book does not go beyond arguing for the entitlement to the CH, though it is undeniable that the next step must be to consider aggregation. That is to say, this book is largely about the 'what' or metric of health justice and not about the 'how' or the rules for distribution. I argue for an entitlement to a sufficient threshold of each CHC that constitutes a health capability, but each of these individual capabilities requires individual assessment in many dimensions. I intend to undertake a separate study of aggregation and health capabilities. As a first step towards that, my current research entails examining the use of capabilities in a non-welfarist approach to economic evaluation of healthcare interventions.

The related topic to aggregation is feasibility. There are both philosophical and practical criticisms about the feasibility of the capability approach. The discussion between Rawls and Sen, at least from Rawls' perspective seems to be less to do with disagreement about capabilities versus primary goods than qualms about feasibility. Rawls thinks that the capabilities approach 'calls for more information than political society can conceivably acquire and sensibly apply' (Rawls, 1999, p.13 fn3). Sen identifies many agreements and disagreements with Rawls beyond feasibility. And, in fact, he argues that the capabilities approach to justice is more feasible or tractable than an ideal, transcendental theory that Rawls advocates (Sen, 2009).

But I leave their disagreements aside. There is then the practical issue of feasibility. It seems that one could say that all the resources expended to find out accurately about the capabilities of people in a country, their causes, constraints, persistence of constraints, levels, distribution patterns, diverse consequences and possible social actions could instead be much better spent by simply giving individuals directly a share of those resources.[1] I think this criticism is right to some extent. When it comes to poverty alleviation, it might be better just to give individuals a share of the money it would take to apply the capabilities approach sufficiently. In its present state the capabilities approach does not have the tools to make it easily operational. But I believe that is simply a question of time. We need to develop better capability measurement tools, try out various pilot studies and do more theoretical work. Some of it has already begun (Chiappero-Martinetti and Roche, 2009), even in relation to health (Coast et al., 2008a, 2008c; Lorgelly et al., 2008; Canoy et al., 2009). Once those tools are developed, the benefits of applying the approach may far outweigh what it would cost to implement. Furthermore, part of feasibility entails that the CH argument and health economics have to be brought together and considered more thoroughly. This is because health economics is king in the domain of health. But that too is also beginning to change (Coast et al., 2008b, 2008c; Mooney, 2009; Smith et al., forthcoming).

There are numerous other aspects about capability theory and health and social justice that were not considered in this book, and hopefully some will be addressed in future research. Such issues include the role of luck in capabilities theory and, therefore, the issues of responsibility and accountability for one's own health and well-being. Then there is the issue of causation. Whether in the natural or social sciences, causation is a difficult concept, and it plays a prominent role in the capabilities approach because the approach is grounded in much empirical research, and in turn, makes various empirical assertions. Without a solid understanding of causality, we will not be able to say with confidence what causes capabilities to go up or down, flourish or fail.

The open acknowledgement of the limitations of the scope of the argument should not, however, take away from what the book does try to achieve. The book advances a concept of health as capability, a theory of causation and distribution of health capability, and it grounds a moral entitlement to health in basic ethical values. It also shows how a right to be healthy can be coherently understood as cluster-right and meta-right. And it shows why a capabilities approach is better than alternative approaches in handling health claims. But as I said in the Introduction, this is only the foundation for being able to assert the centrality of health to the theory and practical evaluation of social justice. There is much more exciting and important work to be done in order to make a human right to the capability to be healthy theoretically sound and practicable.

Notes

Introduction

1 For a compelling overview of global health I recommend the visually illuminating work of the Social and Spatial Inequalities Unit at the University of Sheffield, especially Danny Dorling's slide presentation, 'Making visible global injustice in health: mapping the causes of 57 million deaths' http://sasi.group.shef.ac.uk/presentations/. I also recommend spending time on the website http://www.gapminder.org/ which presents enormous information. Also see the research reports of the Women's Rights Project and the HIV/AIDS Project at Human Rights Watch, the International Center for Research of Women, and the International Women's Health Coalition as well as the most recent World Health Organization's annual World Health Statistics report.

2 An alternative influential account lists the determinants of health and longevity as including biology, environment external to the body, lifestyle and healthcare organization. This model loses a lot of information by combining both physical and social environmental factors together. And it is unclear why the model should separate out healthcare from other external environmental factors. Nevertheless, the model has been influential, at least in Canada, in expanding the public's understanding that health is influenced or determined by more than healthcare. See Lalonde, M. (1974) A New Perspective on the Health of Canadians. In *National Health and Welfare* (ed.), Government of Canada.

3 Rawls writes, 'Other primary goods such as health and vigor, intelligence and imagination, are natural goods; although their possession is influenced by the basic structure, they are not so directly under its control.' However, it is worth noting that the social bases of self-respect, which Rawls considers the most important good of all and is on his list also requires

co-production between the individual and social arrangements. It may simply be that Rawls did not recognize the full extent of social influence on individual health.

4 The two main advocates of the CA, Amartya Sen and Martha Nussbaum, both use the phrase 'capability to be and do'. This has become the standard way of talking about capability (the idea is that the emphasis is on capability rather than on being), and I have therefore used the phrase throughout this volume.

5 See Daniels, N. (1996b) *Justice and Justification: Reflective Equilibrium in Theory and Practice*, Cambridge; New York, Cambridge University Press.

6 For a good example of such a re-fitting of a theory, see Norman Daniels' restatement of his theory in *Just Health*.

7 For example Wolff and De-Shalit argue that the priority of liberty is not always true in Rawlsian justice as he requires the hypothetical social contract to be occurring in an environment of wealth that is adequate to provide for the basic needs of individuals. Thus, they argue that there is a fourth principle of Rawlsian justice, that everyone's basic needs must be satisfied. See Wolff, J. and De-Shalit, A. (2007) *Disadvantage*, Oxford, Oxford University Press [p. 32].

8 I borrow this language from Dale Jamieson, who uses it to describe what he calls the LiveAid conception of famines. What he says about how famines are understood and addressed is, I would argue, not just relevant to famines but more broadly about health and longevity. Jamieson, D. (2005) Duties to the Distant: Aid, Assistance, and Intervention in the Developing World. *Journal of Ethics*, 9, 151.

9 I would argue that this conception of health would constitute a 'non-humiliating' life in the modern world as described in Avishai Margalit's argument or theory for the decent society. But as Margalit expressly does not argue for a conception of justice, I do not pursue his work to any extent in this book. See Margalit, A. (1996) *The Decent Society*, Cambridge, MA; London, Harvard University Press.

10 According to Sen, a meta-right to something, x, can be defined as the right to have policies, p(x), that genuinely pursue the objective of making the right to x realizable.

11 Such a pluralist account is in line with the capabilities approach as any capability can include multiple capabilities. My argument is giving one capability further specification. It would take me away from the present topic to defend a pluralist account of social justice or within a defined domain. I do, however, find much encouragement for advancing this argument in the recent work of Jonathan Wolff and Avner De-Shalit on 'de-clustering' disadvantage. See Wolff and De-Shalit (2007) *Disadvantage*, Oxford, Oxford University Press.

12 Martha Nussbaum has recently published a book on the CA for general readers and instructors of undergraduates. A useful introductory book on the CA has also recently be published on behalf of the Human Develop-

ment and Capability Association. See Deneulin, S. V. and Shahani, L. (2009) *An Introduction to the Human Development and Capability Approach: Freedom and Agency*, London, Earthscan.

13 The German government has begun measuring poverty in terms of capability deprivations. See Bundestag, D. (2008) *Lebenslagen in Deutschland. Der 3. Armuts-und Reichtumsbericht der Bundesregierung*, Cologne, Bundesanzeiger Verlag. President Sarkozy of France appointed the Commission on the Measurement of Economic Performance and Social Progress which included Amartya Sen, and made use of human capabilities as a metric alternative to gross domestic product or GDP per capita. The report can be downloaded from http://www.stiglitz-sen-fitoussi.fr/documents/rapport_anglais.pdf.

14 The background papers to the United Kingdom Equality and Human Rights Commission are thoroughly informed by the capabilities approach. See the background papers, all downloadable at http://www.equalityhumanrights.com/our-job/our-publications/research-reports/. See especially research reports 18 and 31 on developing equality measurement indicators.

15 Marmot Review (2010) *Fair Society, Healthy Lives: Strategic Review of Health Inequalities in England Post 2010*, London, Marmot Review.

16 The Open Left project at the think tank Demos aims to reinvigorate the ideas of the Left political parties, and its director, James Purnell, a former MP, frequently cites Sen and the capabilities approach. For more information see http://www.openleft.co.uk/.

17 Sen's list includes: political freedoms; economic facilities; social opportunities; transparency guarantees; and protective security. Health can fall under protective securities or cut across all the other capabilities as it is needed for other capabilities. Sen, A. (1999a) *Development as Freedom*, New York, Knopf.

1 Health as Capability

1 To account for the health of human beings that do not have recognizable intentionality when they are infants, he offers a modified theory for humans without recognizable intentions. 'Infant I is in health if, and only if, the internal constitution and development of I is such that, given standard adult support, the necessary and jointly sufficient conditions for I's minimal happiness are realized.' Presumably, such a definition would also apply to individuals without full rationality or mental capacities. Nordenfelt, L. (1987) *On the Nature of Health: An Action-Theoretic Approach*, Dordrecht; Boston, D. Reidel Pub. Co.; Kluwer Academic.

2 Causation and Distribution of Health

1 Margaret Whitehead's follow up report in 1987 was also downplayed by the Conservative government, but this report too managed to receive significant public attention. Whitehead, M. (1998) Diffusion of Ideas on

Social Inequalities in Health: A European Perspective. *The Milbank Quarterly*, 76, 469–492, 306. The Whitehead report was then followed by the Acheson Report in 1998 and most recently by the Marmot Review in 2010.

3 The Capabilities Approach

1 See Anderson, E. (1999) What is the Point of Equality? *Ethics*, 109, 287–337; Anderson, E. (2010) Justifying the Capabilities Approach to Justice, in Brighouse, H. and Robeyns, I. (eds) *Measuring Justice. Primary Goods and Capabilities*, Cambridge, Cambridge University Press; Alkire, S. (2002) *Valuing Freedoms: Sen's Capability Approach and Poverty Reduction*, Oxford, Oxford University Press; Robeyns, I. (2003) Sen's Capability Approach and Gender Inequality: Selecting Relevant Capabilities, *Feminist Economics*, 9, 61–92, Alkire, S. (2005a) Needs and Capabilities, *Royal Institute of Philosophy Supplements*, 80, 229–252; Wolff and De-Shalit, *Disadvantage*, Oxford, Oxford University Press; Crocker, D. A. (2008) *Ethics of Global Development: Agency, Capability, and Deliberative Democracy*, Cambridge; New York, Cambridge University Press.
2 See Sen's autobiography written for the 1998 Nobel Prize ceremony. Accessible at http://nobelprize.org/nobel_prizes/economics/laureates/1998/sen-autobio.html.
3 Narayan, D., Chambers, R., Shah, M. K. and Petesch, P. (2000b) *Voice of the Poor. Crying out for Change*, Oxford, published by Oxford University Press for the World Bank; Narayan, D., Chambers, R., Shah, M. K. and Petesch, P. (2000a) *Voice of the Poor. Can Anyone Hear Us?*, Oxford, published by Oxford University Press for the World Bank; Narayan-Parker, D. and Petesch, P. L. (2002) *From Many Lands*, New York; a copublication of Oxford University Press and the World Bank.
4 United Nations Development Programme (1990) *Human Development Report 1990*, New York, Oxford University Press.
5 Burchardt, T. and Vizard, P. (2007) *Definition of Equality and Framework for Measurement: Final Recommendations of the Equalities Review Steering Group on Measurement*, London, CASE, Vizard, P. and Burchardt, T. (2007) *Developing a Capability List: Final Recommendations of the Equalities Review Steering Group on Measurement*, London, CASE.
6 Bundestag, *Lebenslagen in Deutschland. Der 3. Armuts Und Reichtumsbericht Der Bundesregierung* Koln, Bundersanzeiger Verlag.
7 Ostlin, P. and Diderichsen, F. (2001) Equity-Oriented National Strategy for Public Health in Sweden, *Policy Learning Curve Series*. World Health Organization Europe.
8 Stiglitz, J., Sen, A. and Fitoussi, J.-P. (2009a) *The Measurement of Economic Performance and Social Progress Revisited. Reflections and Overview*.
9 The website for the organization is http://www.capabilityapproach.com/.

10 The critique of aggregate or average indicators does not mean that the CA does not value information on populations or social group differences; such information provides information about the capabilities of individuals in the social groups and the success and failures of economic and political institutions.

11 Nussbaum's thresholds seem to be less definitive than what initially appears. While she talks about thresholds defining an ample minimum, when pressed about inequalities above the thresholds, or how thresholds are decided, she seems to argue that justice may require more than sufficient thresholds.

12 In 2004 the United States Supreme Court heard arguments in Tennessee v. Lane where physically disabled plaintiffs argued they were denied access to public services because they could not physically access courtrooms. George Lane, a plaintiff, had to crawl up the courthouse steps in order to appear and defend himself in court while security guards watched and laughed. He was later arrested for failure to appear in court when he refused to crawl or be carried up the stairs at a subsequent hearing. Tennessee v. Lane, 541 U.S. 509 (2004).

13 For an excellent and more even-handed review of utilitarian philosophy and its different branches see Kymlicka, W. (2002) *Contemporary Political Philosophy: An Introduction*, Oxford; New York, Oxford University Press.

14 This problem does not go away for the CA when it endorses capabilities rather than functionings because a set of capabilities is also a certain kind of life. By not identifying a list of capabilities Sen avoids the problem of having to justify a certain kind of life as valuable while Nussbaum expressly identifies the list and provides justification. For further discussion on this see Arneson, R. J. (2000) Perfectionism and Politics. *Ethics*, 111, 37–63. and Sen, A. (2009) *The Idea of Justice*, London, Allen Lane.

15 There is argued to be value in both having options as well as in having meaningful options. This discussion is deferred at this stage because it largely pertains to Sen's conception of the CA. Nussbaum advocates for a particular set of central human capabilities; thus sufficient choice and meaningful breadth is delineated to some extent. She argues that life worthy of the dignity of the human being will have sufficient levels of ten specific capabilities. Sen speaks more abstractly about the value of having choices, and for these choices being valuable or meaningful.

16 These include '(i) basic rights and liberties . . . (ii) freedom of movement and free choice of occupations against a background of diverse opportunities . . . (iii) powers and prerogatives of offices and positions of responsibility . . . (iv) income and wealth . . . (v) the social bases of self-respect'. Rawls, J. (1971) *A Theory of Justice*, Cambridge, MA, Harvard University Press; Rawls, J. (1980) Kantian Constructivism in Moral Theory. *Journal of Philosophy*, 77, 515–572; Rawls, J. (1993) *Political Liberalism*, New York, Columbia University Press.

17 This is reflected in the debate about the instrumental importance of liberties in promoting economic and social well-being, or priority of liberty. Sen, A. (1994) Freedoms and Needs. An Argument for the Primacy of Political Rights. *The New Republic*, 210, 31–38.
18 Bryan Turner also emphasizes the importance of an exit option. See Turner, B. S. (2006) *Vulnerability and Human Rights*, University Park, PA, Pennsylvania State University Press, p. 8.

5 Alternative Approaches

1 The World Health Organization maintains a global reference database of all constraints on health referred to as the International Statistical Classification of Diseases and Related Health Problems, 10th revision.
2 Rights can have a place in consequentialist analysis, as has been argued by Sen. However, such an analysis is not made by health equity advocates. Instead, they advocate absolute rights for instrumental reasons. For an analysis of rights and consequentialist reasoning see Sen, A. (1981c) Rights and Agency, *Philosophy and Public Affairs*, 2, 3–39; Sen, A. (1984) The Right Not to Be Hungry, in Alston, P. and Tomasevski, K. (eds) *The Right to Food*, The Hague, Martinus Nijhoff; Sen, A. (1996a) Legal Rights and Moral Rights: Old Questions and New Problems, *Ratio Juris*, 9, 153–167.
3 For an example of an argument for a moral claim to actions or goods that are not immediately available see Sen's argument for a 'meta-right' or claim of citizens against their government that it must progressively realize economic and social goals. Sen, The Right Not to Be Hungry.
4 See the World Bank's initial public policy recommendations for responding to the spread of HIV/AIDS in developing countries. World Bank (1997) *Confronting Aids: Public Priorities in a Global Epidemic*, New York, Oxford University Press. And for an excellent critical review of the utilitarian health metric, Disability Adjusted Life Years or DALY see Anand, S. and Hanson, K. (1997) Disability-Adjusted Life Years: A Critical Review. *Journal of Health Economics*, 16, 685–702.
5 The criteria for such abrogation of liberties are often that they are constrained by legal means, the least intrusive and time-bound.
6 One of the major drawbacks of Rawls' theory is that when a person's financial needs become very expensive, the theory tries to transform the needs into preferences and thereby absolve any requirements for social provision. And even if there is agreement that there are legitimate, very expensive needs, the theory allows for caps on such expenses because of the prudential reasoning of contractors. Contractors would have an interest in restricting one person from being a large drain on social resources. Pogge, T. (1989) *Realizing Rawls*, Ithaca, NY; London, Cornell University Press; Pogge, T. (1995) 3 Problems with Contractarian-Consequentialist Ways of Assessing Social Institutions, *Social Philosophy and Policy*, 12,

241–266; Pogge, T. (2004) Equal Liberty for All?, *Midwest Studies in Philosophy*, 28, 266.

7 This parallels Cohen's critique of Rawls that though he recognizes that talents are a mix of inheritance and effort, individuals cannot claim their full benefits, but when preferences are also a mix of inheritance and choice, Rawls holds them fully responsible for their tastes. Where there is a mix of individual volition and genetics/unknown reason, how does one identify whether that should fall under choice of brute luck? Cohen, G. A. (1989) On the Currency of Egalitarian Justice, *Ethics*, 99, 906–944; Cohen, G. A. (1997) Where the Action is: On the Site of Distributive Justice. *Philosophy and Public Affairs*, 26, 3–30.

8 This distinction between natural and social sources of inequalities is difficult to sustain especially in light of social determinants of health research. For example, Richard Barker's research connects the impact of a woman's deprivation on her child in-utero and the child's health later in adult life. And Pogge rejects the wholly random nature of natural talents by pointing to the caste and class influences on mating and procreation. Natural endowments are socially affected to some extent.

7   The Capability to be Healthy and Global Justice

1 Readers may be surprised to read that the first Special Rapporterur on the Right to Health states that there is no such thing as a right to health. Committee on Economic, S. A. C. R. 2000. The right to the highest attainable standard of health : 11/08/2000. E/C.12/2000/4. (General Comments). Geneva: United Nations Economic and Social Council.

Conclusion

1 I thank Nomaan Majid for pointing this out to me.

References

Adler, N. E., Boyce, T., Chesney, M. A., Cohen, S., Folkman, S., Kahn, R. L. and Syme, S. L. (1994) Socioeconomic Status and Health. The Challenge of the Gradient. *American Psychologist*, 49, 15–24.

Alkire, S. (2002) *Valuing Freedoms: Sen's Capability Approach and Poverty Reduction*, Oxford, Oxford University Press.

Alkire, S. (2005a) Needs and Capabilities. *Royal Institute of Philosophy Supplements*, 80, 229–252.

Alkire, S. (2005b) Why the Capability Approach? *Journal of Human Development*, 6, 115–133.

Anand, P. (2005) QALYS and Capabilities: A Comment on Cookson. *Health Economics*, 14, 1283–1286.

Anand, P., Hunter, G. and Smith, R. (2005) Capabilities and Well-Being: Evidence Based on the Sen-Nussbaum Approach to Welfare. *Social Indicators Research*, 74, 9–55.

Anand, S. (2002) The Concern for Equity in Health. *Journal of Epidemiology and Community Health*, 56, 485–487.

Anand, S. and Hanson, K. (1997) Disability-Adjusted Life Years: A Critical Review. *Journal of Health Economics*, 16, 685–702.

Anand, S., Peter, F. and Sen, A. (2006) *Public Health, Ethics, and Equity* (paperback), Oxford: Oxford University Press.

Anand, S. and Ravallion, M. (1993) Human Development in Poor Countries: On the Role of Private Incomes and Public Services. *Journal of Economic Perspectives*, 7, 133–150.

Anderson, E. (1999) What is the Point of Equality? *Ethics*, 109, 287–337.

Anderson, E. (2010) Justifying the Capabilities Approach to Justice. In Brighouse, H. and Robeyns, I. (eds) *Measuring Justice. Primary Goods and Capabilities*. Cambridge, Cambridge University Press.

Angell, M. (1993) Caring for Women's Health – What is the Problem? *N Engl J Med*, 329, 271–272.

Antonovsky, A. (1979) *Health, Stress and Coping*, San Francisco; London, Jossey-Bass.

Arneson, R. J. (2000) Perfectionism and Politics. *Ethics*, 111, 37–63.

Arneson, R. J. (2010) Two Cheers for Capabilities. In Brighouse, H. and Robeyns, I. (eds) *Measuring Justice. Primary Goods and Capabilities*, Cambridge, Cambridge University Press.

Arrow, K. (1973) Some Ordinalist–Utilitarian Notes on Rawls' Theory of Justice. *Journal of Philosophy*, 70, 245–263.

Arrow, K. (1951) *Social Choice and Individual Values*, New York, John Wiley and Sons.

Asada, Y. (2005) Assessment of the Health of Americans: The Average Health-Related Quality of Life and its Inequality across Individuals and Groups. *Population Health Metrics*, 3, 7.

Asada, Y. (2007) *Health Inequality: Morality and Measurement*, Toronto; London, University of Toronto Press.

Barker, D. J. (1990) The Fetal and Infant Origins of Adult Disease. *British Medical Journal*, 301, 1111.

Barker, D. J. (1991) The Foetal and Infant Origins of Inequalities in Health in Britain. *J Public Health Med*, 13, 64–68.

Barry, B. (2005) *Why Social Justice Matters*, Cambridge, Polity.

Basu, K., Kanbur, S. M. R. and Sen, A. (2009) *Arguments for a Better World: Essays in Honor of Amartya Sen*, Oxford; New York, Oxford University Press.

Bauman, Z. 2003. *Liquid Love: On the Frailty of Human Bonds*, Cambridge, Polity; Malden, MA: distributed in the USA by Blackwell.

Beitz, C. R. (1975) Justice and International Relations. *Philosophy and Public Affairs*, 4, 360–389.

Beitz, C. R. (1988) Recent International Thought. *International Journal*, 43, 183–204.

Berkman, L. F. and Kawachi, I. O. (2000) *Social Epidemiology*, New York, Oxford University Press.

Bhargava, R. (2008) *Individualism in Social Science: Forms and Limits of a Methodology*, Oxford, Oxford University Press.

Biggs, B., King, L., Basu, S. and Stuckler, D. (2010a) Is Wealthier Always Healthier? The Impact of National Income Level, Inequality, and Poverty on Public Health in Latin America. *Social Science and Medicine*.

Black, D., Morris, J. N., Smith, C., Townsend, P. and Whitehead, M. (1992) *Inequalities in Health. The Black Report. The Health Divide*, London, Penguin Books.

Blaxter, M. (2010) *Health*, Cambridge, Polity.

Bloom, D. E. and Canning, D. (2007) Commentary: The Preston Curve 30 Years On: Still Sparking Fires. *International Journal of Epidemiology*, 36, 498–499.

Boorse, C. (1975) On the Distinction between Disease and Illness. *Philosophy and Public Affairs*, 5, 49–68.

Boorse, C. (1976a) What a Theory of Mental Health Should Be. *Journal for the Theory of Social Behaviour*, 6, 61–84.

Boorse, C. (1976b) Wright on Functions. *Philosophical Review*, 85, 70–86.

Boorse, C. (1977) Health as a Theoretical Concept. *Philosophy of Science*, 44, 542–573.

Boorse, C. (1997) A Rebuttal on Health. In Humber, J. M. and Almeder, R. F. (eds) *Biomedical Ethics Reviews. What is Disease?* Clifton, NJ, Humana Press.

Boorse, C. (2002) A Rebuttal on Functions. In Ariew, A., Cummins, R. and Perlman, M. (eds) *Functions: New Essays in the Philosophy of Psychology and Biology*. Oxford, Oxford University Press.

Boorse, C. (2004) Four Recent Accounts of Health. *Conference on Medicine and Metaphysics*. New York, University of Buffalo.

Braveman, P. (2006) Health Disparities and Health Equity: Concepts and Measurement. *Annual Review of Public Health*, 27, 167–194.

Braveman, P. and Gruskin, S. (2003) Defining Equity in Health. *J Epidemiol Community Health*, 57, 254–258.

Braveman, P., Krieger, N. and Lynch, J. (2000) Health Inequalities and Social Inequalities in Health. *Bull World Health Organ*, 78, 232–234; discussion 234–235

Braveman, P., Starfield, B., Geiger, H. J. and Murray, C. J. L. (2001) World Health Report 2000: How it Removes Equity from the Agenda for Public Health Monitoring and Policy. *Bulletin of the World Health Organization*, 323, 678–681.

Bristol, N. (2008) William H. Stewart. *Lancet*, 372, 110.

Brock, D. W. (1995) Quality of Life Measures in Healthcare and Medical Ethics. In Nussbaum, M. C. and Sen, A. (eds) *Quality of Life*. New York, Oxford University Press.

Brock, D. W. (2002) The Separability of Health and Well-Being. In Murray, C. J. L., Salomon, J. A., Mathers, C. D. and Lopez, A. D. (eds) *Summary Measures of Population Health. Concepts, Ethics, Measurement and Applications*. Geneva, World Health Organization.

Brock, G. (2005) Needs and Global Justice. In Reader, S. (ed.) *The Philosophy of Need*. Cambridge, Cambridge University Press.

Broome, J. (2006) *Weighing Lives*, Oxford, Clarendon.

Brown, G. W. and Held, D. (2010) *The Cosmopolitanism Reader*, Cambridge, Polity.

Deutscher Bundestag (2008) *Lebenslagen in Deutschland. Der 3. Armuts-und Reichtumsbericht Der Bundesregierung*, Cologne, Bundesanzeiger Verlag.

Burchardt, T. (2004) Capabilities and Disability: The Capabilities Framework and the Social Model of Disability. *Disability and Society*, 19, 735–751.

Burchardt, T. and Vizard, P. (2007) *Definition of Equality and Framework for Measurement: Final Recommendations of the Equalities Review Steering Group on Measurement*, London, CASE.

Campbell, D. (2010) Top GP Condemns Britons for Recklessly Neglecting Their Health. *Observer*. London.

Caney, S. (2005) *Justice Beyond Borders: A Global Political Theory*, Oxford, Oxford University Press.

Canoy, M., Lerais, F. and Schokkaert, E. (2009) Applying the Capability Approach to Policy-Making: The Impact Assessment of the EU-Proposal on Organ Donation. *Journal of Socio-Economics*, 39, 391–399.

Cartwright, N. (2007) *Hunting Causes and Using Them: Approaches in Philosophy and Economics*, Cambridge, Cambridge University Press.

Cassel, J. (1976) The Contribution of the Social Environment to Host Resistance: The Fourth Wade Hampton Frost Lecture. *American Journal of Epidemiology*, 104, 107–123.

Chiappero-Martinetti, E. and Roche, J. M. (2009) Operationalization of the Capability Approach, from Theory to Practice: A Review of Techniques and Empirical Applications. In Chiappero-Martinetti, E. (ed.) *Debating Global Society. Reach and Limits of the Capability Approach*. Milan, Fondazione Giangiacomo Feltrinelli; Grafica Sipiel.

Childress, J., Faden, R., Gaare, R., Gostin, L., Kahn, J., Bonnie, R., Kass, N., Mastroianni, A., Moreno, J. and Nieburg, P. (2002) Public Health Ethics: Mapping the Terrain. *Journal of Law, Medicine, and Ethics*, 30, 170–178.

Coast, J., Flynn, T. N., Natarajan, L., Sproston, K., Lewis, J., Louviere, J. J. and Peters, T. J. (2008a) Valuing the Icecap Capability Index for Older People. *Social Science and Medicine*, 67, 874–882.

Coast, J., Smith, R. and Lorgelly, P. (2008b) Should the Capability Approach Be Applied in Health Economics? *Health Economics*, 17, 667–670.

Coast, J., Smith, R. D. and Lorgelly, P. (2008c) Welfarism, Extra-Welfarism and Capability: The Spread of Ideas in Health Economics. *Social Science and Medicine*, 67, 1190–1198.

Coburn, D. (2004) Beyond the Income Inequality Hypothesis: Class, Neo-Liberalism, and Health Inequalities. *Soc Sci Med*, 58, 41–56.

Cohen, G. A. (1989) On the Currency of Egalitarian Justice. *Ethics*, 99, 906–944.

Cohen, G. A. (1997) Where the Action is: On the Site of Distributive Justice. *Philosophy and Public Affairs*, 26, 3–30.

Commission on Social Determinants of Health (2008) Closing the Gap in a Generation: Health Equity through Action on the Social Determinants of Health. Final Report of the Commission on Social Determinants of Health. Geneva, World Health Organization.

Cookson, R. (2005) QALYs and the Capability Approach. *Health Economics* 14(8): 817–829.

Cribb, A. (2001) Reconfiguring Professional Ethics: The Rise of Managerialism and Public Health in the UK National Health Service. *HEC Forum*, 13, 111–124.

Cribb, A. (2005) *Health and the Good Society: Setting Healthcare Ethics in Social Context*, Oxford, Clarendon Press.

Crocker, D. A. (2008) *Ethics of Global Development: Agency, Capability, and Deliberative Democracy*, Cambridge; New York, Cambridge University Press.

Daniels, N. (1985) *Just Healthcare*, Cambridge; New York, Cambridge University Press.

Daniels, N. (1996a) Equality of What: Welfare, Resources, or Capabilities? *Justice and Justification: Reflective Equilibrium in Theory and Practice*, Cambridge; New York, Cambridge University Press.

Daniels, N. (1996b) *Justice and Justification: Reflective Equilibrium in Theory and Practice*, Cambridge; New York, Cambridge University Press.

Daniels, N. (2007) Just Health - a Population Perspective (unpublished manuscript). Cambridge.

Daniels, N. (2008) *Just Health: Meeting Health Needs Fairly*, Cambridge; New York, Cambridge University Press.

Daniels, N. (2010) Capabilities, Opportunity, and Health. In Brighouse, H. and Robeyns, I. (eds) *Measuring Justice. Primary Goods and Capabilities*, Cambridge, Cambridge University Press.

Daniels, N., Kennedy, B. P. and Kawachi, I. (1999) Why Justice is Good for Our Health: The Social Determinants of Health Inequalities. *Daedalus*, 128, 215–251.

Deaton, A. (2011) What Does the Empirical Evidence Tell Us About the Injustice of Health Inequalities? Princeton, Center for Health and Wellbeing.

DeJong, J. (2006) Capabilities, Reproductive Health and Well-Being. *Journal of Development Studies*, 42, 1158–1179.

Deneulin, S. V. and Shahani, L. (2009) *An Introduction to the Human Development and Capability Approach: Freedom and Agency*, London, Earthscan.

Dolan, P. (2000) The Measurement of Health-Related Quality of Life for Use in Resource Allocation Decisions in Healthcare. In Culyer, A. J. and Newhouse, J. P. (eds) *Handbook of Health Economics*. Amsterdam; Oxford, Elsevier.

Dolan, P., Shaw, R., Tsuchiya, A. and Williams, A. (2005) QALY Maximisation and People's Preferences: A Methodological Review of the Literature. *Health Economics*, 14, 197–208.

Drèze, J. and Sen, A. K. (1989) *Hunger and Public Action*, Oxford, Clarendon.

Dworkin, R. (1993) Justice in the Distribution of Healthcare. *McGill Law Journal*, 38, 883–898.

Dworkin, R. (2000) *Sovereign Virtue: The Theory and Practice of Equality*, Cambridge, MA, Harvard University Press.

Epstein, S. (1996) *Impure Science: Aids, Activism, and the Politics of Knowledge*, Berkeley, University of California Press.

Evans, R. G. and Stoddart, G. L. (1990) Producing Health, Consuming Healthcare. *Soc Sci Med*, 31, 1347–1363.

Evans, T., Whitehead, M., Diderichsen, F., Bhuiya, A. and Wirth, M. (eds) (2001) *Challenging Inequities in Health: From Ethics to Action*, Oxford; New York, Oxford University Press.

Farley, T. A. (2009) Reforming Healthcare or Reforming Health? *Am J Public Health*, 99, 588–590.

Field, S. (2010) Don't Take Offence If We Lecture You on How to Stay Alive and Healthy. *Observer*. London.

Fleurbaey, M. (2008) *Fairness, Responsibility, and Welfare*, Oxford; New York, Oxford University Press.

Francis, L. P., et al. (2005) How Infectious Diseases Got Left out- and What This Omission Might Have Meant for Bioethics. *Bioethics*, 19, 307–322.

Gakidou, E., Murray, C. J. L. and Frenk, J. (2000) A Framework for Measuring Health Inequality. *Bulletin of the World Health Organization*, 78, 42–54.

Gore, C. (1997) Irreducibly Social Goods and the Informational Basis of Amartya Sen's Capability Approach. *Journal of International Development*, 9.

Hofrichter, R. (2003) *Health and Social Justice: A Reader on the Politics, Ideology, and Inequity in the Distribution of Disease*, San Francisco, Jossey-Bass.

Huppert, F. A. and Baylis, N. (2004) Well-Being: Towards an Integration of Psychology, Neurobiology and Social Science. *Philos Trans R Soc Lond B Biol Sci*, 359, 1447–1451.

Huppert, F. A., Baylis, N. and Keverne, B. (2004) Introduction: Why Do We Need a Science of Well-Being? *Philos Trans R Soc Lond B Biol Sci*, 359, 1331–1332.

Illich, I. (1974) Medical Nemesis. *Lancet*, 1, 918–921.

Jamieson, D. (2005) Duties to the Distant: Aid, Assistance, and Intervention in the Developing World. *Journal of Ethics*, 9, 151.

Jones, C. (1999) *Global Justice: Defending Cosmopolitanism*, Oxford [England]; New York, Oxford University Press.

Kamm, F. M. (1993) *Morality, Mortality. Volume I: Death and Whom to Save from it* New York; Oxford, Oxford University Press.

Kass, N. (2001) An Ethics Framework for Public Health. *American Journal of Public Health*, 91, 1776–1782.

Kass, N. E. (2004) Public Health Ethics: From Foundations and Frameworks to Justice and Global Public Health. *J Law Med Ethics*, 32, 232–242, 190.

Kawachi, I., Daniels, N. and Robinson, D. E. (2005) Health Disparities by Race and Class: Why Both Matter. *Health Affairs*, 24, 343–352.

Kawachi, I., Kennedy, B. P. and Wilkinson, R. G. (eds) (1999) *The Society and Population Health Reader. Income Inequality and Health*, New York, The New Press.

Kelly, M., Morgan, A., Ellis, S., Younger, T., Huntley, J. and Swann, C. (2010) Evidence Based Public Health: A Review of the Experience of the National Institute of Health and Clinical Excellence (Nice) of Developing Public Health Guidance in England. *Soc Sci Med*.

Khushf, G. (1987) What is at Issue in the Debate About Concepts of Health. *On the Nature of Health: An Action-Theoretic Approach*. Dordrecht; Boston, D. Reidel Pub. Co.

Kittay, E. (1997) Human Dependency and Rawlsian Equality. In Meyers, D. T. (ed.) *Feminists Rethink the Self.* Boulder, Westview Press.

Kreisler, H. (2002) Conversations with History: Michael Marmot. Berkeley, Institute of International Studies, UC Berkeley.

Krieger, N. (1994) Epidemiology and the Web of Causation: Has Anyone Seen the Spider? *Soc Sci Med,* 39, 887–903.

Krieger, N. (2001) Historical Roots of Social Epidemiology: Socioeconomic Gradients in Health and Contextual Analysis. *Int J Epidemiol,* 30, 899–900.

Krieger, N. and Davey Smith, G. (2004) 'Bodies Count,' and Body Counts: Social Epidemiology and Embodying Inequality. *Epidemiol Rev,* 26, 92–103.

Krieger, N., Rehkopf, D. H., Chen, J. T., Waterman, P. D., Marcelli, E. and Kennedy, M. (2008) The Fall and Rise of US Inequities in Premature Mortality: 1960–2002. *PLoS Med,* 5, e46.

Kuklys, W. (2005) *Amartya Sen's Capability Approach: Theoretical Insights and Empirical Applications,* Berlin; New York, Springer.

Kymlicka, W. (1989) *Liberalism, Community, and Culture,* Oxford, Clarendon Press.

Kymlicka, W. (2002) *Contemporary Political Philosophy: An Introduction,* Oxford; New York, Oxford University Press.

Lafaille, R. and Fulder, S. (1993) *Towards a New Science of Health,* London; New York, Routledge.

Lalonde, M. (1974) A New Perspective on the Health of Canadians. In *National Health and Welfare* (ed.), Government of Canada.

Larmore, C. E. (1987) *Patterns of Moral Complexity,* Cambridge; New York, Cambridge University Press.

Larmore, C. E. (1996) *The Morals of Modernity,* Cambridge [England]; New York, Cambridge University Press.

Law, I. and Widdows, H. (2008) Conceptualising Health: Insights from the Capability Approach. *Healthcare Analysis,* 16, 303–314.

Levins, R. and Lewontin, R. C. (1985) *The Dialectical Biologist,* Cambridge, MA, Harvard University Press.

Levins, R. and Lopez, C. (1999) Toward an Ecosocial View of Health. *Int J Health Serv,* 29, 261–293.

Lin, C. C., Rogot, E., Johnson, N. J., Sorlie, P. D. and Arias, E. (2003) A Further Study of Life Expectancy by Socioeconomic Factors in the National Longitudinal Mortality Study. *Ethnicity and Disease,* 13, 240–247.

Lobb, A. (2009) Healthcare and Social Spending in OECD Nations. *Am J Public Health,* 99, 1542–1544; author reply 1544.

Lorgelly, P., Lorimer, K., Fenwick, E. and Briggs, A. (2008) The Capability Approach: Developing an Instrument for Evaluating Public Health Interventions. Glasgow, University of Glasgow. Section of Public Health and Health Policy.

Macinko, J. and Starfield, B. (2001) The Utility of Social Capital in Research on Health Determinants. *The Milbank Quarterly,* 79, 387–427, IV.

Macintyre, S. (1997) The Black Report and Beyond: What Are the Issues? *Soc Sci Med*, 44, 723–745.

Macmahon, B., Pugh, T. F. and Ipsen, J. (1960) *Epidemiologic Methods*, Boston, Little, Brown and Company.

Marmot Review (2010) *Fair Society, Healthy Lives: Strategic Review of Health Inequalities in England Post 2010*, London, Marmot Review.

Majumdar, M. and Subramanian, S. (2001) Capability Failure and Group Disparities: Some Evidence from India for the 1980s. *Journal of Development Studies*, 37.

Mann, J. M. (1996) Health and Human Rights. *British Medical Journal*, 312, 924–925.

Mann, J. M. (1997) Medicine and Public Health, Ethics and Human Rights. *Hastings Center Report*, 27, 6–13.

Mann, J. M., Gostin, L., Gruskin, S., Brennan, T., Lazzarini, Z. and Fineberg, H. V. (1994) Health and Human Rights. *Health and Human Rights*, 1, 6–23.

Mann, J. M., Tarantola, D. and Netter, T. W. (1992) *Aids in the World*, Cambridge, MA, Harvard University Press.

Margalit, A. (1996) *The Decent Society*, Cambridge, MA; London, Harvard University Press.

Marmor, J. (1972) Homosexuality – Mental Illness or Moral Dilemma? *Int J Psychiatry*, 10, 114–117.

Marmot, M. (1976) Facts, Opinions and Affaires Du Coeur. *American Journal of Epidemiology*, 103, 519–526.

Marmot, M. (2004a) Dignity and Inequality. *Lancet*, 364, 1019–1021.

Marmot, M. (2005) Social Determinants of Health Inequalities. *Lancet*, 365, 1099–1104.

Marmot, M. (2006) Health in an Unequal World: Social Circumstances, Biology and Disease. *Clinical Medicine*, 6, 559–572.

Marmot, M., Ryff, C. D., Bumpass, L. L., Shipley, M. and Marks, N. F. (1997) Social Inequalities in Health: Next Questions and Converging Evidence. *Soc Sci Med*, 44, 901–910.

Marmot, M. G. (2004b) *Status Syndrome: How Your Social Standing Directly Affects Your Health and Life Expectancy*, London, Bloomsbury.

Marmot, M. G. and Brunner, E. (1999) Social Organization, Stress, and Health. In Marmot, M. G. and Wilkinson, R. G. (eds) *Social Determinants of Health*. Oxford; New York, Oxford University Press.

Marmot, M. G., Fuhrer, R., Ettner, S. L., Marks, N. F., Bumpass, L. L. and Ryff, C. D. (1998) Contribution of Psychosocial Factors to Socioeconomic Differences in Health. *The Milbank Quarterly*, 76, 403–448, 305.

Marmot, M. G., Rose, G., Shipley, M. and Hamilton, P. J. (1978) Employment Grade and Coronary Heart Disease in British Civil Servants. *J Epidemiol Community Health*, 32, 244–249.

Marmot, M. G., Shipley, M. J., Hemingway, H., Head, J. and Brunner, E. J. (2008) Biological and Behavioural Explanations of Social Inequalities in Coronary Heart Disease: The Whitehall II Study. *Diabetologia*, 51, 1980–1988.

Marmot, M. G., Siegrist, J. and Theorell, T. (1999) Health and the Psychosocial Environment at Work. In Marmot, M. G. and Wilkinson, R. G. (eds) *Social Determinants of Health.* Oxford; New York, Oxford University Press.

Marmot, M. G. and Syme, S. L. (1976) Acculturation and Coronary Heart Disease in Japanese-Americans. *American Journal of Epidemiology*, 104, 225–247.

Marmot, M. G. and Wilkinson, R. G. (1999) *Social Determinants of Health*, Oxford; New York, Oxford University Press.

Mooney, G. (2005) Communitarian Claims and Community Capabilities: Furthering Priority Setting? *Soc Sci Med*, 60, 247–255.

Mooney, G. H. (2009) *Challenging Health Economics*, Oxford, Oxford University Press.

Murray, C. J. (1996) Rethinking Dalys. In Murray, C. J. L. and Lopez, A. (eds) *The Global Burden of Disease: A Comprehensive Assessment of Mortality and Disability from Diseases, Injuries, and Risk Factors in 1990 and Projected to 2020.* Boston, MA, Harvard School of Public Health on behalf of the World Health Organization and the World Bank.

Murray, C. J., Gakidou, E. E. and Frenk, J. (1999a) Health Inequalities and Social Group Differences: What Should We Measure? *Bull World Health Organ*, 77, 537–543.

Murray, C. J. L. (1994) Quantifying the Burden of Disease: The Technical Basis for Disability-Adjusted Life Years. *Bulletin of the World Health Organization*, 72, 429–445.

Murray, C. J. L., Gakidou, E. E. and Frenk, J. (1999b) Health Inequalities and Social Group Differences: What Should We Measure? *Bulletin of the World Health Organization*, 77, 537–543.

Murray, C. J. L. and Lopez, A. (1996) *The Global Burden of Disease: A Comprehensive Assessment of Mortality and Disability from Diseases, Injuries, and Risk Factors in 1990 and Projected to 2020.* Boston, MA, Harvard School of Public Health on behalf of the World Health Organization and the World Bank.

Murray, C. J. L., Michaud, M. C., Mckenna, M. and Marks, J. (1998) U.S. Patterns of Mortality by County and Race: 1965–1994. *Harvard Center for Population and Development Studies.* Cambridge, MA.

Nagel, T. (1997) Justice and Nature. *Oxford Journal of Legal Studies*, 17, 303–321.

Nagel, T. (2005) The Problem of Global Justice. *Philosophy and Public Affairs*, 33.

Narayan-Parker, D. and Petesch, P. L. (2002) *From Many Lands*, New York; [Great Britain], a copublication of Oxford University Press and the World Bank.

Narayan, D., Chambers, R., Shah, M. K. and Petesch, P. (2000a) *Voice of the Poor. Can Anyone Hear Us?*, Oxford, published by Oxford University Press for the World Bank.

Narayan, D., Chambers, R., Shah, M. K. and Petesch, P. (2000b) *Voice of the Poor. Crying out for Change*, Oxford, published by Oxford University Press for the World Bank.

Navarro, V. (1993) *Dangerous to Your Health: Capitalism in Healthcare*, New York, Monthly Review Press.

Navarro, V. and Shi, L. (2001) The Political Context of Social Inequalities and Health. *Soc Sci Med*, 52, 481–491.

Nordenfelt, L. (1987) *On the Nature of Health: An Action-Theoretic Approach*, Dordrecht; Boston, D. Reidel Pub. Co.; Kluwer Academic.

Nordenfelt, L. (1993) On the Notions of Disability and Handicap. *International Journal of Social Welfare*, 2, 17–24.

Nordenfelt, L. (2000) *Action, Ability and Health: Essays in the Philosophy of Action and Welfare*, Dordrecht, Kluwer Academic Publishers.

Nordenfelt, L. (2007) Establishing a Middle-Range Position in the Theory of Health: A Reply to My Critics. *Medicine, Healthcare and Philosophy*, 10, 29–32.

Nordenfelt, L., Khushf, G. and Fulford, K. W. M. (2001) *Health, Science, and Ordinary Language*, Amsterdam, Rodopi.

Nordenfelt, L. and Lindahl, B. I. B. (1984) *Health, Disease, and Causal Explanations in Medicine*, Dordrecht; Boston, Reidel; Kluwer Academic Publishers.

Nuffield Council on Bioethics (2007) Public Health: Ethical Issues. London, Nuffield Council on Bioethics.

Nussbaum, M. (2001) Political Objectivity. *New Literary History*, 32, 883–906.

Nussbaum, M. C. (1987) Nature, Function, and Capability: Aristotle on Political Distribution. *World Institute for Development Economics Research Working Papers*. Helsinki.

Nussbaum, M. C. (1999) *Sex and Social Justice*, New York, Oxford University Press.

Nussbaum, M. C. (2000a) Aristotle, Politics, and Human Capabilities: A Response to Antony, Arneson, Charlesworth, and Mulgan. *Ethics*, 111, 102–140.

Nussbaum, M. C. (2000b) *Women and Human Development: The Capabilities Approach*, Cambridge; New York, Cambridge University Press.

Nussbaum, M. C. (2006) *Frontiers of Justice: Disability, Nationality, Species Membership*, Cambridge, MA; London, The Belknap Press of Harvard University Press.

Nussbaum, M. C. (2011) *Creating Capabilities: The Human Development Approach*, Cambridge, MA; London, Belknap.

Nussbaum, M. C., Glover, J. and World Institute for Development Economics Research. (1995) *Women, Culture, and Development: A Study of Human Capabilities*, New York, Oxford University Press.

Nussbaum, M. C. and Sen, A. K. (1993) *The Quality of Life*, New York, Clarendon Press; Oxford University Press.

O'Connor, T. and Sandis, C. (2010) *A Companion to the Philosophy of Action*, Oxford, Wiley-Blackwell.

O'Neill, O. (1993) Justice, Gender and International Relations. In Nussbaum, M. and Sen, A. (eds) *The Quality of Life*. Oxford, Clarenden Press.

O'Neill, O. (2000) *Bounds of Justice*, Cambridge, Cambridge University Press.

O'Neill, O. (2002a) *Autonomy and Trust in Bioethics: The Gifford Lectures, University of Edinburgh, 2001*, Cambridge, Cambridge University Press.

O'Neill, O. (2002b) Public Health or Clinical Ethics: Thinking Beyond Borders. *Ethics and International Affairs*, 16, 35–45.

O'Neill, O. (2002c) *A Question of Trust*, Cambridge, Cambridge University Press.

O'Neill, O. (2004a) 'Global Justice: Whose Obligations?' *The Ethics of Assistance: Morality and the Distance Needy*, Chatterjee, Deen K (Ed), 242, 259. Cambridge, Cambridge University Press.

O'Neill, O. (2004b) Informed Consent and Public Health. *Philosophical Transactions of the Royal Society B: Biological Sciences*, 359, 6.

O' Neill, O. (2010) The Idea of Justice. Amartya Sen (Book Review). *Journal of Philosophy*, 107, 384–388.

Omran, A. R. (1971) The Epidemiologic Transition. A Theory of the Epidemiology of Population Change. *The Milbank Quarterly*, 49, 509–538.

Ostlin, P. and Diderichsen, F. (2001) Equity-Oriented National Strategy for Public Health in Sweden. *Policy Learning Curve Series*. World Health Organization Europe.

Parfit, D. (1997) Equality and Priority. *Ratio-New Series*, 10, 202–221.

Peter, F. and Evans, T. (2001) Ethical Dimensions of Health Equity. In Evans, T., Whitehead, M., Diderichsen, F., Bhuiya, A. and Wirth, M. (eds) *Challenging Inequities in Health: From Ethics to Action*. Oxford; New York, Oxford University Press.

Pettit, P. (2001) Symposium on Amartya Sen's Philosophy: 1 Capability and Freedom: A Defence of Sen. *Economics and Philosophy*, 17, 1–20.

Pierik, R. and Robeyns, I. (2007) Resources Versus Capabilities: Social Endowments in Egalitarian Theory. *Political Studies*, 55, 133–152.

Pogge, T. (1989) *Realizing Rawls*, Ithaca, NY; London, Cornell University Press.

Pogge, T. (1995) 3 Problems with Contractarian-Consequentialist Ways of Assessing Social Institutions. *Social Philosophy and Policy*, 12, 241–266.

Pogge, T. (2001) *Global Justice*, Oxford, Blackwell.

Pogge, T. (2002a) Can the Capability Approach Be Justified? *Philosophical Topics*, 30, 167–228.

Pogge, T. (2002b) *World Poverty and Human Rights: Cosmopolitan Responsibilities and Reforms*, Cambridge; Malden, MA, Polity.

Pogge, T. (2004) Equal Liberty for All? *Midwest Studies In Philosophy*, 28, 266.

Pogge, T. (2005) Real World Justice. *Journal of Ethics*, 9, 29–53.

Pogge, T. (2010) A Critique of the Capability Approach. In Brighouse, H. and Robeyns, I. (eds) *Measuring Justice. Primary Goods and Capabilities*. Cambridge, Cambridge University Press.

Posner, R. A. 1992. *Sex and Reason*. Cambridge, MA; London, Harvard University Press.

Powers, M. and Faden, R. R. (2008) *Social Justice: The Moral Foundations of Public Health and Health Policy*, New York; Oxford, Oxford University Press.

Preston, S. H. (1975) Changing Relation between Mortality and Level of Economic Development. *Population Studies – A Journal of Demography*, 29, 231–248.

Preston, S. H. (2007) Response: On 'the Changing Relation between Mortality and Level of Economic Development'. *International Journal of Epidemiology*, 36, 502–503.

Pritchett, L. and Summers, L. H. (1996) Wealthier is Healthier. *Journal of Human Resources*, 31, 841–868.

Putnam, R. D. (2000) *Bowling Alone: The Collapse and Revival of American Community*, New York, Simon and Schuster.

Putnam, R. D., Leonardi, R. and Nanetti, R. (1993) *Making Democracy Work: Civic Traditions in Modern Italy*, Princeton, NJ, Princeton University Press.

Qizilbash, M. (1997) Pluralism and Well-Being Indices. *World Development*, 25, 2009–2026.

Rawls, J. (1971) *A Theory of Justice*, Cambridge, MA, Harvard University Press.

Rawls, J. (1980) Kantian Constructivism in Moral Theory. *Journal of Philosophy*, 77, 515–572.

Rawls, J. (1993) *Political Liberalism*, New York, Columbia University Press.

Rawls, J. (1999) *The Law of Peoples*, Cambridge, MA, Harvard University Press.

Rawls, J. and Freeman, S. R. (2007) *Lectures on the History of Political Philosophy*, Cambridge, MA, Belknap Press of Harvard University Press.

Rawls, J. and Kelly, E. (2001) *Justice as Fairness: A Restatement*, Cambridge, MA, Harvard University Press.

Reid, E. (1992) Gender, Knowledge and Responsibility. Issues Paper No. 10. New York, UNDP HIV and Development Programme.

Robert Wood Johnson Foundation Commission to Build a Healthier America (2009) Beyond Healthcare: New Directions to a Healthier America. Recommendations from the Robert Wood Johnson Foundation Commission to Build a Healthier America. Princeton, NJ, Robert Wood Johnson Foundation.

Roberts, M. and Reich, M. (2002) Ethical Analysis in Public Health. *Lancet*, 359, 1055–1059.

Robeyns, I. (2002) In Defence of Amartya Sen. *Post-Autistic Economics Review*.

Robeyns, I. (2003) Sen's Capability Approach and Gender Inequality: Selecting Relevant Capabilities. *Feminist Economics*, 9, 61–92.

Robeyns, I. (2005a) The Capability Approach: A Theoretical Survey. *Journal of Human Development*, 6, 93–114.

Robeyns, I. (2005b) Selecting Capabilities for Quality of Life Measurement. *Social Indicators Research*, 74, 191–215.

Robeyns, I. (2006) The Capability Approach in Practice. *Journal of Political Philosophy*, 14, 351–376.

Robeyns, I. (2011) *The Capability Approach* [Online]. Stanford: Stanford University. Available: http://plato.stanford.edu/archives/sum2011/entries/capability-approach/ [Accessed 19 April 2011].

Roemer, J. E. (1993) A Pragmatic Theory of Responsibility for the Egalitarian Planner. *Philosophy and Public Affairs*, 22, 144–166.

Rogot, E., Sorlie, P. D. and Johnson, N. J. (1992) Life Expectancy by Employment Status, Income, and Education in the National Longitudinal Mortality Study. *Public Health Reports*, 107, 457–461.

Rose, G. (1985) Sick Individuals and Sick Populations. *Int J Epidemiol*, 14, 32–38.

Rothman, K. J., Adami, H. O. and Trichopoulos, D. (1998) Should the Mission of Epidemiology Include the Eradication of Poverty? *Lancet*, 352, 810–813.

Rothman, K. J., Greenland, S. and Lash, T. L. (2008) *Modern Epidemiology*, Philadelphia, Wolters Kluwer Health/Lippincott Williams and Wilkins.

Ruger, J. P. (2010) *Health and Social Justice*, Oxford, Oxford University Press.

Saleeby, P. W. (2007) Applications of a Capability Approach to Disability and the International Classification of Functioning, Disability and Health (ICF) in Social Work Practice. *Journal of Social Work in Disability and Rehabilitation*, 6, 217–232.

Sandel, M. J. (1996) *Democracy's Discontent: America in Search of a Public Philosophy*, Cambridge, MA, Belknap Press of Harvard University Press.

Sangiovanni, A. (2007) Global Justice, Reciprocity, and the State. *Philos Public Aff*, 35, 3–39.

Saracci, R. (2010) Introducing the History of Epidemiology. In Olsen, J. (ed.) *Teaching Epidemiology*. New York, Oxford University Press.

Schramme, T. (2007) A Qualified Defence of a Naturalist Theory of Health. *Medicine, Healthcare and Philosophy*, 10, 11–17.

Segall, S. (2009) *Health, Luck, and Justice*, Princeton, NJ; Woodstock, Princeton University Press.

Sen, A. (1976) Famines as Failures of Exchange Entitlements. *Economic and Political Weekly*, 11.

Sen, A. (1977) Starvation and Exchange Entitlements: A General Approach and its Application to the Great Bengal Famine. *Cambridge Journal of Economics*, 1, 33–59.

Sen, A. (1981a) Ingredients of Famine Analysis: Availability and Entitlements. *The Quarterly Journal of Economics*, 96, 433–464.

Sen, A. (1981b) *Poverty and Famines: An Essay on Entitlement and Deprivation*, Oxford, New York, Clarendon Press; Oxford University Press.

Sen, A. (1981c) Rights and Agency. *Philosophy and Public Affairs*, 2, 3–39.

Sen, A. (1982a) *Choice, Welfare, and Measurement*, Cambridge, MA, MIT Press.

Sen, A. (1982b) Equality of What? *Choice, Welfare, and Measurement*. Cambridge, MA, MIT Press.

Sen, A. (1983) Poor, Relatively Speaking. *Oxford Economic Papers*, 35, 153–169.

Sen, A. (1984) The Right Not to Be Hungry. In Alston, P. and Tomasevski, K. (eds) *The Right to Food*. The Hague, Martinus Nijhoff.

Sen, A. (1985a) *Commodities and Capabilities*, Amsterdam, North-Holland.

Sen, A. (1985b) Well-Being, Agency and Freedom. The Dewey Lectures 1984. *Journal of Philosophy*, 82, 169–221.

Sen, A. (1988) Freedom of Choice. Concept and Content. *European Economic Review*, 32, 269–294.

Sen, A. (1992a) *Inequality Reexamined*, Cambridge, MA, Harvard University Press.

Sen, A. (1992b) Objectivity, Health and Policy. In Das Gupta, M., Chen, L. C. and Krishnan, T. N. (eds) *Health and Development in India*. New Delhi, Oxford University Press.

Sen, A. (1993) The Economics of Life and Death. *Scientific American*, 268, 40–47.

Sen, A. (1994) Freedoms and Needs. An Argument for the Primacy of Political Rights. *The New Republic*, 210, 31–38.

Sen, A. (1995) Mortality as an Indicator of Economic Success and Failure. *1st Innocenti Lecture of UNICEF*. Florence, Italy.

Sen, A. (1996a) Legal Rights and Moral Rights: Old Questions and New Problems. *Ratio Juris*, 9, 153–167.

Sen, A. (1996b) On the Status of Equality. *Political Theory*, 24, 394–400.

Sen, A. (1997) *Resources, Values, and Development*, Cambridge, MA, Harvard University Press.

Sen, A. (1998a) Health Achievement and Equity: External and Internal Perspectives. In Anand, S., Peter, F. and Sen, A. K. (eds) *Global Health Equity Initiative; Public Health, Ethics and Equity*. Harvard University, Oxford:.

Sen, A. (1998b) Why Health Equity? In Anand, S., Peter, F. and Sen, A. K. (eds) *Global Health Equity Initiative; Public Health, Ethics and Equity*, Harvard University, Oxford.

Sen, A. (1999a) *Development as Freedom*, New York, Knopf.

Sen, A. (1999b) Economic Progress and Health. In Leon, D. A. and Walt, G. (eds) *Poverty, Inequality, and Health*, London, Oxford.

Sen, A. (1999c) Economics and Health. *Lancet*, 354 Suppl, SIV20.

Sen, A. (1999d) Health in Development. *Bull World Health Organ*, 77, 619–623.

Sen, A. (2000) The Discipline of Cost-Benefit Analysis. *Journal of Legal Studies*, 29, 931–952.

Sen, A. (2001b) Health Equity: Perspectives, Measurability, and Criteria. In Evans, T., Whitehead, M., Diderichsen, F., Bhuiya, A. and Wirth, M. (eds) *Challenging Inequities in Health: From Ethics to Action*. Oxford; New York, Oxford University Press.

Sen, A. (2001c) Symposium on Amartya Sen's Philosophy: Reply. *Economics and Philosophy*, 17, 51–66.

Sen, A. (2002a) Health: Perception Versus Observation. *British Medical Journal*, 324, 860–861.

Sen, A. (2002b) Response to Commentaries. *Studies in Comparative International Development*, 37, 78–86.

Sen, A. (2002c) Why Health Equity? *Health Economics*, 11, 659–666.

Sen, A. (2004a) Capabilities, Lists, and Public Reason: Continuing the Conversation. *Feminist Economics*, 10, 77–80.

Sen, A. (2004b) Disability and Justice. *2004 World Bank International Disability Conference*. Washington, DC.

Sen, A. (2004c) Elements of a Theory of Human Rights. *Philos Public Aff*, 32, 315–355.

Sen, A. (2005) Open and Closed Impartiality. In Kuper, A. (ed.) *Global Responsibilities: Who Must Deliver on Human Rights?* New York, Routledge.

Sen, A. (2006) What Do We Want from a Theory of Justice? *Journal of Philosophy*, 103, 215–238.

Sen, A. (2007) The World of Smoking Guns. *Tob Control*, 16, 59–63.

Sen, A. (2009) *The Idea of Justice*, London, Allen Lane.

Sen, A. (2010) The Place of Capability in a Theory of Justice. In Brighouse, H. and Robeyns, I. (eds) *Measuring Justice. Primary Goods and Capabilities*. Cambridge, Cambridge University Press.

Sen, A. (2011) Learning from Others. *Lancet*, 377, 200–201.

Sen, A. and Williams, B. A. O. (eds) (1982) *Utilitarianism and Beyond*, Cambridge; New York, Cambridge University Press.

Shapiro, I. and Brilmayer, L. (eds) (1999) *Global Justice*, New York, New York University Press.

Siegrist, J. and Marmot, M. (2004) Health Inequalities and the Psychosocial Environment – Two Scientific Challenges. *Soc Sci Med*, 58, 1463–1473.

Singer, P. (1972) Famine, Affluence, and Morality. *Philosophy and Public Affairs*, 1, 229–243.

Singer, P. (2002) A Response to Martha Nussbaum. http://www.utilitarian.net/singer/by/20021113.htm.

Singh-Manoux, A. (2003) Psychosocial Factors and Public Health. *J Epidemiol Community Health*, 57, 553–556; discussion 554–555.

Smith, R., Coast, J., Lorgelly, P., Al-Janabi, H. and Venkatapuram, S. (forthcoming) The Capabilities Approach. In Jones, A. M. (ed.) *The Elgar Companion to Health Economics*. Cheltenham, Edward Elgar.

Sontag, S. (1978) *Illness as Metaphor*, New York, Farrar, Straus and Giroux.

Sorlie, P., Rogot, E., Anderson, R., Johnson, N. J. and Backlund, E. (1992) Black-White Mortality Differences by Family Income. *Lancet*, 340, 346–350.

Stewart, F. (2005) Groups and Capabilities. *Journal of Human Development*, 6, 185–204.

Stewart, F. and Deneulin, S. (2002) Amartya Sen's Contribution to Development Thinking. *Studies in Comparative International Development*, 37, 61–70.

Stiglitz, J., Sen, A. and Fitoussi, J.-P. (2009) *The Measurement of Economic Performance and Social Progress Revisited. Reflections and Overview.*

Stoller, R. J., Marmor, J., Bieber, I., Gold, R., Socaride.Cw, Green, R. and Spitzer, R. L. (1973) Symposium - Should Homosexuality Be in APA Nomenclature. *American Journal of Psychiatry*, 130, 1207–1216.

Subramanian, S. V. and Kawachi, I. (2004) Income Inequality and Health: What Have We Learned So Far? *Epidemiologic Reviews*, 26, 78–91.

Susser, M. (1985) Epidemiology in the United States after World War II: The Evolution of Technique. *Epidemiologic Reviews*, 7, 147–177.

Susser, M. (1994a) The Logic in Ecological: I. The Logic of Analysis. *Am J Public Health*, 84, 825–829.

Susser, M. (1994b) The Logic in Ecological: II. The Logic of Design. *Am J Public Health*, 84, 830–835.

Susser, M. (1999) Should the Epidemiologist Be a Social Scientist or a Molecular Biologist? *International Journal of Epidemiology*, 28, S1019-S1022.

Susser, M. and Susser, E. (1996a) Choosing a Future for Epidemiology: I. Eras and Paradigms. *Am J Public Health*, 86, 668–673.

Susser, M. and Susser, E. (1996b) Choosing a Future for Epidemiology: II. From Black Box to Chinese Boxes and Eco-Epidemiology. *Am J Public Health*, 86, 674–677.

Syme, S. L. (1996) Rethinking Disease: Where Do We Go from Here? *Ann Epidemiol*, 6, 463–468.

Syme, S. L. (1998) Social and Economic Disparities in Health: Thoughts About Intervention. *The Milbank Quarterly*, 76, 493–505.

Syme, S. L. and Balfour, J. L. (1997) Explaining Inequalities in Coronary Heart Disease. *Lancet*, 350, 231–232.

Szasz, T. S. (1960) The Myth of Mental Illness. *American Psychologist*, 15, 113–118.

Szreter, S. (1984) The Genesis of the Registrar-General's Social Classification of Occupations. *British Journal of Sociology*, 35, 522–546.

Szreter, S. (1997) Economic Growth, Disruption, Deprivation, Disease, and Death: On the Importance of the Politics of Public Health for Development. *Population and Development Review*, 23, 693–.

Szreter, S. (2002) The State of Social Capital: Bringing Back in Power, Politics, and History. *Theory and Society*, 31, 573–621.

Taurek, J. M. (1977) Should the Numbers Count? *Philosophy and Public Affairs*, vol. 6, Summer 1977.

Taylor, C. (1992) *The Ethics of Authenticity*, Cambridge, MA, Harvard University Press.

Temkin, L. S. (1993) *Inequality*, New York; Oxford, Oxford University Press.

Terzi, L. (2010) What Metric of Justice for Disabled People? Capability and Disability. In Brighouse, H. and Robeyns, I. (eds) *Measuring Justice. Primary Goods and Capabilities.* Cambridge, Cambridge University Press.

Thaler, R. H. and Sunstein, C. R. (2008) *Nudge: Improving Decisions About Health, Wealth, and Happiness*, New Haven, Yale University Press.

Thomson, J. J. (1990) *The Realm of Rights*, Cambridge, MA, Harvard University Press.

Tilly, C. (1999) *Durable Inequality*, Berkeley, University of California Press.

Trostle, J. A. (2004) *Epidemiology and Culture*, Cambridge; New York, Cambridge University Press.

Turner, B. M. (2004) *The New Medical Sociology: Social Forms of Health and Illness*, New York, W.W. Norton.

Turner, B. S. (2006) *Vulnerability and Human Rights*, University Park, PA, Pennsylvania State University Press.

United Nations Development Programme (1990) *Human Development Report 1990*, New York, Oxford University Press.

Vagero, D. and Illsley, R. (1995) Explaining Health Inequalities. Beyond Black and Barker – a Discussion of Some Issues Emerging in the Decade Following the Black Report. *European Sociological Review*, 11, 219–241.

Venkatapuram, S. (2006) Culture and Epidemiology. Book Review. *Medicine, Healthcare and Philosophy*, 10, 97–99.

Venkatapuram, S. and Marmot, M. (2009) Epidemiology and Social Justice in Light of Social Determinants of Health. *Bioethics*, 23, 78–89.

Vizard, P. (2006) *Poverty and Human Rights: Sen's 'Capability Perspective' Explored*, Oxford, Oxford University Press.

Vizard, P. and Burchardt, T. (2007) *Developing a Capability List: Final Recommendations of the Equalities Review Steering Group on Measurement*, London, CASE.

Walzer, M. (1983) *Spheres of Justice: A Defense of Pluralism and Equality*, New York, Basic Books.

Wasserman, D. (2006) Disability, Capability, and Thresholds for Distributive Justice. In Kaufman, A. (ed.) *Capabilities Equality: Basic Issues and Problems*. New York; London, Routledge.

Weed, D. (1996) Epistemology and Ethics in Epidemiology. In Coughlin, S. S. and Beauchamp, T. L. (eds) *Ethics and Epidemiology*. New York, Oxford University Press.

Weed, D. (2001) Theory and Practice in Epidemiology. *Annals of the New York Academy of Sciences*, 954, 52–62.

Weed, D. L. and Mckeown, R. E. (1998) Epidemiology and Virtue Ethics. *International Journal of Epidemiology*, 27, 343–349.

Weed, D. L. and Mckeown, R. E. (2001) Ethics in Epidemiology and Public Health I. Technical Terms. *Journal of Epidemiology and Community Health*, 55, 855–857.

Whitehead, M. (1990) *The Concepts and Principles of Equity in Health*. Copenhagen, World Health Organization Regional Office for Europe.

Whitehead, M. (1992) The Concepts and Principles of Equity and Health. *International Journal of Health Services*, 22, 429–445.

Whitehead, M. (1998) Diffusion of Ideas on Social Inequalities in Health: A European Perspective. *The Milbank Quarterly*, 76, 469–492, 306.

Wikler, D. (2004) Personal and Social Responsibility for Health. In Anand, S., Peter, F. and Sen, A. K. (eds) *Public Health, Ethics and Equity*, Oxford; New York, Oxford University Press.

Wilkinson, R. G. (1992) Income Distribution and Life Expectancy. *British Medical Journal*, 304, 165–168.

Wilkinson, R. G. (1996) *Unhealthy Societies: The Afflictions of Inequality*, London, Routledge.

Wilkinson, R. G. (1997) Socioeconomic Determinants of Health. Health Inequalities: Relative or Absolute Material Standards? *British Medical Journal*, 314, 591–595.

Wilkinson, R. G. (2000) The Need for an Interdisciplinary Perspective on the Social Determinants of Health. *Health Economics*, 9, 581–583.

Wilkinson, R. G. and Pickett, K. (2009) *The Spirit Level: Why More Equal Societies Almost Always Do Better*, London, Allen Lane.

Wilkinson, R. G. and Pickett, K. E. (2006) Income Inequality and Population Health: A Review and Explanation of the Evidence. *Soc Sci Med*, 62, 1768–1784.

Williams, A. (2002) Dworkin on Capability. *Ethics*, 113, 23–39.

Wolff, J. and De-Shalit, A. (2007) *Disadvantage*, Oxford, Oxford University Press.

World Bank (1997) *Confronting Aids: Public Priorities in a Global Epidemic*, New York, Oxford University Press.

World Health Organization (2000) *Health Systems: Improving Performance*, Geneva.

World Health Organization (2001) International Classification of Functioning, Disability and Health (ICF). Geneva, World Health Organization.

World Health Organization (2007) International Statistical Classification of Diseases and Related Health Problems. 10th revision. Version of 2007. Geneva, World Health Organization.

World Health Organization and Commission on Social Determinants of Health (2008) Closing the Gap in a Generation. Health Equity through Action on the Social Determinants of Health. Geneva, World Health Organization.

Index